Disclaimer

This book contains advice and information relating to healthcare.
It is intended as a reference volume only; it is not intended to be
used as a medical manual. The information given here is designed
to help you make informed decisions about your health. It is not
intended as a substitute for any treatment that may be prescribed
by your doctor. If you know or suspect that you have a health
problem, it is recommended that you seek your physician's advice
before embarking on any medical program or treatment. All efforts
have been made to ensure the accuracy of the information
contained in this book as of the date of publication. The publisher
and author disclaim liability for any medical outcomes that may
occur as a result of applying the methods suggested in this book.

The Savage Diet. Copywrite 2024

D1738600

Copywrite Page

ISBN 979-8-9923552-0-8

Chapter 5: Your Savage Journey

Section 1: In the Shadow of Time

Section 2: Awakening Your Awareness

Section 3: Adopting The Savage Principles

Chapter 6: Unlocking Nutrient Potential: Mastering Advanced Bioavailability Section 1: Advanced Nutritional Tactics

Section 2: Optimizing Nutrient Bioavailability

Section 3: Short Chain Fatty Acids

Section 4: Nutrient Cycling

Section 5: The Benefits of Emulating Ancient Patterns

Section 6: Strategic Fasting

Chapter 7: The Use of Oils, Wheat, and Dairy (and why we do not use them) Section 1: Omega 6 vs Omega 3 Ratios

Section 2: Wheat as We Knew It and Where Did it Go?

Section 3: The Perfect Storm…..How This Affects Our Health Section 4: Globalization

Section 5: Convenience

Part III: Reversing Modern Illnesses with The Savage Diet

Chapter 8: The Savage Recipes

Section 1: Cooking Tips

Chapter 11: Your Savage Journey

Section 1: Diet Wars: Keto, Paleo, and Mediterranean – Which Best Supports Your Gut?

Section 2: Gut Health and Keystone Microbes

Section 3: The Importance of Gut Health for Immunity and Digestion Section 4: Fermented Foods and Natural Probiotics in The Savage Diet Section 5: Gut Diversity and Brain Health

Section 6: Gut Microbes and the Stress Response

Section 7: Cognitive Function and Memory

Section 8: Gut Health and the Blood-Brain Barrier

Part VII: The Scientific Backbone

Introduction

I began my career as an EMT at the age of 16, becoming the youngest person in my home state to achieve that distinction in the early 1970s. I then joined the U.S. Navy, making history as the first woman to receive the Wet Crewman designation as a Search and Rescue Corpsman. After retiring, I became a licensed Naturopathic Physician and have been practicing in this role for the past 16 years. In my work as a Naturopathic Physician, I have dedicated countless hours to studying our diet, researching other societies, and exploring the numerous diseases we face today; this is the first culmination of that knowledge.

In the whispered hush of dawn's first light, through the tangled brush, a hunter's sight, crouched low, eyes fierce with primal might, a caveman stalks through the shadows' bite.

With spear in hand, forged sharp and true, he moves with the breath of the morning dew, the peccary nears, its fate unbeknown, in the dance of survival, the wild has grown.

A swift thrust forth, as quick as thought, where survival's lesson is keenly taught, the spear finds hold beneath the thick hide, and the peccary falls in the morning tide.

Victory's bitter, life's price paid, on the forest floor, the beast is laid, a tribe will feast as night descends, In the cycle of life, where the wild bends.

The quote below sparked my journey to write this book.

(Medicare (MCM 2251.3)

"Care that seeks to prevent disease, promote health, and prolong and enhance the quality of life, is not considered medically necessary, and therefore not payable."

In a world brimming with dietary fads and quick-fix health trends, "The Savage Diet" stands out as a beacon of fundamental truth, calling us back to the origins of human nutrition. This book is not merely a guide; it is a compelling invitation to reevaluate and reconstruct our daily eating habits based on the diet our bodies were originally designed to thrive on.

As we navigate the 21st century, the challenges to our health continue to grow in complexity. Processed foods, misleading dietary advice, and a sedentary lifestyle have distanced us from the vitality and wellness that should be our birthright. The number of people on the internet trying to sell information for quick weight-loss programs is astronomical. In response, "The Savage Diet" offers a call to embrace the wisdom of our ancestors, who flourished on whole, unprocessed foods rich in nutrients and free from modern additives.

The brilliance of "The Savage Diet" lies not only in its advocacy for a return to a more natural way of eating but in its deep understanding of why our modern diet has led us astray. This book bridges the gap between ancient dietary wisdom and contemporary nutritional science, offering a well-researched, compelling argument that the secret to good health is hidden in plain sight—in the foods that our ancestors hunted, gathered, and consumed with respect for nature's cycles.

I have meticulously crafted a guide that is both informative and transformative. Drawing upon extensive research and personal experiences, I do not just tell you what to eat; I explain why these choices can change your life, improve your health, and align you more closely with the natural world. The book goes beyond the plate, exploring how the principles of The Savage Diet can affect everything from your energy levels and digestion to your sleep patterns and mental health. As you restore your body to health, you will notice your hormones returning to more stable levels, your mood will improve, and you will no longer feel the sugar cravings you once experienced. Your energy, which you thought was a thing of the past, will feel like it did when you were in your 20s.

While many Americans live longer than their parents, they do not necessarily live healthier or happier lives. Lifestyle diseases such as obesity, diabetes, and heart disease are on the rise as the Standard American Diet (SAD) has largely become dominated by processed foods high in sugar, fat and chemicals.

This shift in diet can be partly attributed to changing agricultural systems that have prioritized yields and shelf life over nutrition.

Besides lacking nutrition, industrial farming impacts human health both directly and indirectly through exposure to potentially toxic chemicals and environmental pollutants.

Our medical system is overwhelmed, trying to treat chronic diseases with pharmaceutical interventions.

Meanwhile, conventional farming practices rely on harmful inputs that compromise human health and

prioritize crops low in nutritional value. With rising cancer rates and autoimmune diseases worldwide, we need a new approach to enhancing health.

We are more disconnected from our food and the natural rhythms of life than ever before. This was not always the case. For millions of years, our ancestors thrived by consuming what nature provided—whole, nutrient-dense foods that supported their physical, mental, and emotional well-being. They lived in harmony with the land, their bodies, and the seasons, and they enjoyed better health as a result. They always had the possibility of having to fight a saber-toothed tiger, but their health was good. We examine the Dawn of the Savage Diet, reconnecting with our primal way of eating, and contrast it with the modern, processed food-centric Downfall of the Savage Life, which has led us to the chronic diseases we experience today. The book will then guide you through Embracing the Savage Shift, offering practical advice on transitioning from the Standard American Diet to a more nourishing, ancestral way of eating.

As we delve deeper into the Savage Diet, we will explore the building blocks of health, focusing on the importance of nutrient-dense foods and their role in our overall well-being. We also dive into Gut Health and the Keystone Microbes, revealing how our digestive health impacts everything from immune function to mental clarity. The use of oils, wheat and dairy are discussed, guiding you in choosing the healthiest options while avoiding harmful ingredients. The book will highlight how The Savage Diet can be a powerful tool in the reversal of chronic diseases, offering hope and healing for those dealing with conditions like diabetes, autoimmune diseases, and other imbalances of the body. Living an ancestral life goes beyond diet, which is why we include practical tips on Living the Ancestral Life, featuring exercises and recipes that are both simple, and effective. We provide real-world strategies for maintaining this lifestyle even in our busy, modern world. Finally, we will compare Savage vs Modern diets, showing you how a return to ancestral eating can restore balance, strength and vitality. Through each chapter, The Savage Diet is not just a guide to eating, but a complete lifestyle transformation, empowering you to reconnect with your primal health and unlock your full potential.

Every page of this book is infused with passion, making The Savage Diet both a practical guide to healthier living and a philosophical exploration of our relationship with food. It challenges us to make mindful choices, respect our bodies, and honor the environment. This book is essential reading for anyone seeking to reclaim their health, understand their body's natural needs, and cultivate a sustainable lifestyle that promotes wellness and a deeper, richer understanding of life closer to nature.

As you turn these pages, prepare to embark on a journey that is about much more than a diet. It is a voyage back to the very essence of human well-being. Welcome to The Savage Diet—a path to a healthier, more vibrant you, guided by the enduring wisdom of our ancestors.

Part 1: Awakening the Savage Within

Chapter 1: The Dawn of Time

Section 1: The Foundation of the Savage Diet

I invite you to journey back in time with me to rediscover the eating habits that fueled our ancestors. In The Savage Diet, we will learn practices deeply intertwined with the rhythms of nature and our human biology. We will explore the core philosophy behind The Savage Diet, highlighting why this approach is more than just a nutritional plan—it's a return to the eating patterns and lifestyle that our ancestors thrived on. By choosing to follow this path, you're not only changing what you eat; you're embracing a new way of life—sleeping at night and rising in the morning, the Caveman way. You will learn how our ancestors used drums in spiritual and healing ceremonies. You will experience the changes within yourself by harnessing the body's natural connection to the environment, rising with the warm glow of the sun, and then falling

asleep with the colder, darker nights. There are many rituals that support and promote health and wellness, and we will delve into this in much more detail.

I want you to embrace the eating habits of our prehistoric forebears and examine their lifestyles with a modern twist. I advocate for a back-to-basics approach that bridges the gap between the ancient Caveman and the breakneck pace of modern life. In this journey, I aim to unlock a sustainable and healthy approach to nutrition and lifestyle.

I invite you to imagine yourself transported 20,000 years into the past, wrapped in furs and foraging for food. Picture the firelight dancing on your face as you prepare your next meal—a meal rich in nutrients your body was designed to thrive on. I'll help you bring this mindset into the modern day.

Understanding the foundation of The Savage Diet is the first step in reclaiming your health. But to truly thrive, we must go beyond dietary habits and awaken something deeper within us: the primal instincts that make us human.

Chapter 2: Dawn of the Savage Diet – Returning to the Ancestral Plate Section 1: A Shift In Time

We are starting our journey in the Upper-Paleolithic time period which was also known as the Old Stone Age, this spanned from about 2.6 million years ago to roughly 10,000 years ago when the Neolithic period began. During this time, the Earth was approaching the last Ice Age. There were dramatic climatic shifts and also a challenging landscape that was difficult, but provided for our ancestors. This is essential for understanding the period that we are dealing with.

However, human presence in what is now known as the United States dates back only to the latter part of the Paleolithic period, which was approximately 15,000 -20,000 years ago, and since this is the most widely accepted archaeological evidence we have, we will go with it.

I want to take us back to approximately 20,000 years ago, where our journey to enlightenment will begin.

Our Earth was vastly different at that time, living as hunter-gatherers was not an option, this was our survival. Our lives were intimately connected to nature in a way that modern civilizations have largely forgotten. Understanding their way of life will shed light on the dietary principles that will form the core of The Savage Diet. Twenty thousand years ago, certain practices were essential for survival. They were not choices but necessities to remain safe and healthy. Today, there are many of the same practices that abound now and have become popularized by the internet, but they are disjointed. For example, on a weekend we may go back to nature. We will pack up and take all of the conveniences of home (and maybe take our home as an RV) and we will take with us everything to eat; all of the processed food items, e.g. hotdogs, cheddar cheese, spaghetti, etc and then go back on Monday and feel as if we have communed with nature. Which in today's lifestyle may be the best that some can do, but I propose a different path for those that are adventuresome and have a wild heart.

It is generally accepted that the more indigenous people of the world increasingly need to learn from us, the more advanced and highly educated people we have become, and therefore, we will teach the noneducated people or the traditional people. I believe it is the accumulated wisdom of our ancestors that we need to pay more attention to if we want to live a long and healthy life. Rather than seeing ourselves as more advanced, we should approach ancestral wisdom with humility and curiosity. Their ways of life holds timeless truths about health, resilience, and connection to nature—truths we risk losing in our pursuit of convenience.

We were primitive 20,000 years ago, and we have attained such a stature that we have forgotten where we came from. Today, we no longer migrate with the seasons or walk miles to find food, but incorporating

more movement into our daily lives—even simple acts like walking or hiking—can restore a part of this ancestral rhythm.

As we begin our journey, we discover that we are a nomadic people, moving with the seasons to follow the animal migrations as well as the plant growth cycles. This constant movement required endurance and strength, shaping the robust skeletal structure and muscle development of our ancestors—qualities we can strive to emulate through functional, natural movement today.

This was the rhythm of our lives, the constant movement was not just a quest for food, but a flow of life that kept us physically fit and deeply attuned to the environment. We are part of a small band or tribe of people who over the course of time migrated to what is the mid-western United States. Although there is little evidence of us having been present at this time, it is likely we existed in small groups and left little evidence behind, but we would have hunted and used the area for seasonal migration of the megafauna that was present. We would have gathered the edible plants, roots, and berries, and we would have hunted the mammoth and bison that were present.

This was during the height of the Ice Age (the late Pleistocene period), and it would have been dramatically different from today. It would have had sharp climatic conditions, more glacial landscapes, and would have also had the presence of megafauna. The megafauna that were present during that period refers to the large animals in the region, in our case because of the fossils that are found we know that we would have had a mix of many different types of animals, such as mammoths, mastodons, giant ground sloths, scary saber-toothed tigers and short-faced bears. These large animals provided not only sustenance but also a wide range of essential nutrients that supported survival in harsh conditions. They competed with us for their food, and they were crucial to our survival, providing food, clothing, and materials for tools and shelter.

The weather is cold and more volatile due to the presence of glacial periods, which were part of the last Ice Age. During this time, it is important to understand the United States was not like it is now, much of North America was covered in glaciers, leaving only pockets of habitable land. Survival demanded resilience and adaptability to the harsh, ever-changing environment. As a savage, you find yourself in a very wild and desolate area after migrating across the Bering Land Bridge (Beringia), which connected Siberia to Alaska and followed southward migration routes either along the Pacific coast or through an ice-free corridor that opened up as the glaciers receded. Our ancestors consumed what the land provided: fresh, unprocessed, nutrient-dense foods. They moved constantly, rested when needed, and lived in tune with the cycles of the earth. These principles form the foundation of The Savage Diet and can guide us toward a healthier, more balanced way of living today.

There were few groups of people able to spend any length of time in any one area, simply because the animals graze and would move on to greener pastures. There were not just grazing animals present, there were also animals who would eat berries and succulent plants and would be in direct competition for food sources. There is a mixture of arid deserts, high plateaus, and mountain ranges with a cooler and wetter climate than we enjoy today. By the end of the Ice Age, the climate was changing rapidly, which altered the habitats and food availability.

Section 2: A Day in the Life of the Caveman (Paleolithic Experience Perspective) Join me as we envision your first day as a "caveman." Your given name is Ekon. This name, while foreign to you today, was typical for the time, carrying with it a meaning of strength and resilience. As you were born, you exhibited such vigor and cried out with such a powerful cry, that this prompted the shaman to declare that you would be called "Ekon". The Shaman foresaw that you would be a strong warrior and a great hunter, which would be vital to the tribe's survival. There was a ceremony following your birth, which was significant for the whole tribe as this was your welcoming into the community. There was symbolism to this, during the celebration of your birth, you were passed over a fire and as the warmth

bathed your skin as you were passed from warrior to warrior, the rhythmic chant of the tribe echoed under the night sky. The Shaman's touch was cool, his sacred water a blessing on your newborn forehead As Ekon, your name sets you apart, and with this - certain expectations within the tribe. You are looked upon as a future leader, a central figure in hunts and tribal defense. As you have grown, the ties to the community's needs and their spiritual beliefs, along with your achievements are seen as reflections of your name's power. Your name is not just a tag to call you by, but it is a mantle that you carry, embodying the strength and resilience for the survival and prosperity of your tribe. It connects you with your tribe and directs your role within the tribe and will be passed down through the years as told by your actions around the fires and celebrations at night.

So, close your eyes and imagine that you are Ekon, living 20,000 years ago. Far enough from our present society timeline to not have any hint of modern convenience. You have your spear and a knife involving a combination of natural resourcefulness and inherited knowledge that you shaped by hours of honing it to the sharpness it has. There is meaning behind everything, your spear and knife are not just instruments, they are connections to your tribe's traditions and technological ingenuity. The tools you use are the lifeline of survival and the skills it took to craft them have been passed down from generation to generation. In Ekon's world, your spear and knife serve as the essential lifeline of survival.

Section 3: The Hunt

The sun rose slowly over the horizon, stretching its first rays across the dry grasslands of the ancient savannah. The cool morning breeze whispered through the trees, carrying with it the distant calls of animals stirring from sleep. In the midst of this vast and untamed world, a lone figure crouched, scanning the landscape for the first meal of the day. This was no ordinary morning. It was another day in the endless rhythm of survival.

Your stomach growls, telling you are hungry and it is time to find something to eat. The winter is approaching as the wind blows colder, you know you would need to go out to get food to have more for everyone to eat.

Ekon and his group of hunters moved with the silence of a shadow, their feet barely rustling the dense underbrush. His tribe's survival hinged on hunts like these. Winter was approaching, and the meat and fat would sustain them through the lean, cold months when game was scarce. He climbed a ridge, his eyes scanning the verdant expanse spread beneath him. The land was alive with the rustle of small creatures and the distant calls of birds, but it was the tracks in the mud by a stream that caught his attention—a fresh set of hoof prints, deeper than those of a deer, they were from an elk, and not alone; it moved with its herd. Ekon leads the hunting party, tracking hoof prints through thickets and damp earth, deeper into the elk's domain. His heart beat in rhythm with his steps, each thud a drum of war against the silence of the hunt.

Hours passed as they tracked the herd, the sun climbing overhead, filtering through the dense canopy in shafts of light. The ground beneath their feet is soft, muffling their steps. They crouched low, using the terrain as cover. Then, ahead in a clearing, he saw them—grazing quietly, unaware of the danger at their flanks. The elk graze, their massive antlers swaying as they tug at the tough grass. The hunters pause, waiting for the flankers to drive the elk toward them. Ekon signals with a silent hand motion, his eyes locked on the lead bull elk—a massive animal with an impressive rack of antlers. Its size makes it a prized target, offering meat, hides, and tools that the tribe will need to survive. Ekon crouched low, blending into the underbrush, his grip tightening around the shaft of his spear. He chose his target: a robust elk separated slightly from the rest, its hide dark and muddy. Ekon measured the wind, felt the earth beneath him, and waited for the moment when all became still. With a burst of energy, he sprinted forward, his feet pounding the ground, his presence now known to the herd. The herd startled, but not quickly enough. Ekon's spear flew through the air, a swift, sure motion honed by years of survival. The strike was true, hitting the elk in the flank, the flint tip sinking deep. The animal stumbled, then fell, its

cries echoing through the forest, calling its herd to scatter. Ekon approached cautiously, his respect for the animal evident in his somber expression. With another quick motion, he ended its suffering, a prayer escaping his lips to honor its spirit.

As Ekon and his hunters prepared the elk for the journey back to camp, he reflected on the hunt. Each venture into the wilderness was a dance with fate, a test of wills between man and nature. Today, he was victorious, but the humility of the hunt never left him. By the time Ekon and the others returned to the tribe, the sun was setting, casting long shadows over the land. The children rushed to greet him, their laughter countering the day's grim tasks. His partner's relief was palpable as she helped him with his burden. While you had gone to hunt the elk, others went out and gathered more berries, seeds and wild plants. These were placed on the fire and while others cooked the elk over the fire, the rich, smoky scent filled the air, mingling with the earthy aroma of crushed berries and roasted seeds. The crackle of flames and the soft hum of conversation created a sense of warmth and unity within the tribe. This one meal was most likely the main meal of the day and you enjoyed it while telling story around the fire. As it gets dark fairly early in the cave you lay down to go to sleep. Your sleep patterns are closely aligned with the natural light cycles. Ekon felt a deep, satisfying fatigue. It was more than the weariness of the body—it was the contentment of having sustained his tribe, of fulfilling his role in the great, unending cycle of life and survival. With the stars emerging above in the firelight, Ekon's story of the hunt became a part of his tribe's lore, whispered to the beat of a drum, a tale of courage, skill, and the eternal respect between hunter and hunted. This is the balance we've lost in modern life—but it's a balance we can begin to restore, one mindful step at a time

You are nomadic so you will only be in this area for a few more weeks before moving on. Then, just as the buffalo and the woolly mammoth migrate, to follow the grass, you follow them. Each day you will hunt and forage for food. In the late afternoon times or in the early evening, you may make a tool while others are cooking and preparing meat. Each member of the tribe had a role, with skills that were honed from early childhood to complement the group's needs.

Ask yourself, how would it feel to rely entirely on your skills and instincts to feed your family? To feel the satisfaction of earning your meal through effort and precision?

Ekon's tribe lived in harmony with the seasons, eating what they hunted and gathered. In contrast, modern humans are surrounded by convenience, yet we've lost the connection to our food and environment. By incorporating ancestral practices into our daily lives, we can reclaim a piece of this balance.

Section 4: The Essence of Survival

In modern life, we rarely face the physical challenges that Ekon's tribe did, yet these struggles created a profound connection to their food, their environment, and their community. Reclaiming even small elements of this lifestyle—through movement, mindful eating, or rituals of gratitude—can restore a sense of purpose and vitality. Today, convenience often dictates what we eat, and processed foods dominate the shelves. But even small steps—like choosing whole, unprocessed foods or sitting down to eat without distractions—can bring us closer to the nourishing simplicity of Ekon's world. Seasonal eating—

consuming fruits, vegetables, and proteins that are naturally available at certain times of the year—

connects us to the earth's cycles. In today's world, this might look like visiting a local farmer's market or researching what's in season in your area. By eating seasonally, we not only nourish our bodies but also support sustainable farming practices.

In our ancient world, food was not readily available. It was something that had to be earned. A successful hunt requires patience, endurance, and respect for the natural world. His diet, shaped by necessity, was diverse but seasonal. Some days he feasted on fresh game—meat rich in fats and nutrients, the fuel that powered his active life. On other days, he foraged the earth for roots, nuts, seeds, and fruits, each bite a gift from the wild. There were no processed grains or refined sugars. No snacks to munch on mindlessly.

Food was simple, yet profoundly nourishing, offering everything needed to sustain strength, endurance, and clarity of mind. It was a way of eating born not from convenience but from alignment with the rhythms of the land—a diet that mirrored the cycles of the seasons, the migrations of animals, and the rise and fall of the sun. Food was simple yet profoundly nourishing, sustaining strength, endurance, and clarity of mind. Ekon's meals were not measured in calories or macros, but in survival—did the meal sustain him through the next hunt? Did it keep his muscles strong and his mind sharp? Did it nourish his body enough to fend off illness and injury? This was food as it was meant to be: fuel, medicine, and a sacred connection to the earth that provided it.

Section 5: The Legacy of the Savage Diet

The story of Ekon is not just a tale of the past—it is a reflection of what we have lost in the modern world.

Our ancestors understood that food was sacred, that it required effort and respect, and that what we eat shapes who we are. The Savage Diet is a call to return to this wisdom, to align our eating habits with the natural rhythms of the earth, and to nourish ourselves in a way that sustains both body and spirit. The food that they obtained was shared communally, and meals were often preceded by a moment of silence or a whispered prayer of gratitude to the animal or plant that had given its life. This act of mindfulness deepened their connection to the earth and to each other – a practice that modern life has largely forgotten.

Ekon's tribe wasted nothing, honoring the life of every plant and animal they consumed. By adopting more sustainable practices—such as reducing food waste or choosing ethical, locally sourced ingredients—we can carry forward this respect for the earth and its resources.

Food was not just fuel for Ekon—it was an experience shared with his tribe, a source of joy, gratitude, and connection. In our busy lives, we can rediscover this by slowing down, savoring meals, and sharing them with loved ones. Eating with intention can transform a simple meal into a moment of connection and celebration.

In the upcoming chapters, we will explore how the principles of The Savage Diet can be applied to modern life. We will learn to eat with intention, move purposefully, and live in harmony with the natural world. Just as Ekon thrived by listening to the land and following the rhythms of life, we, too, can rediscover the path to health and vitality.

As you continue reading, I encourage you to start small: take a moment for mindfulness before your next meal, spend a few minutes outside each day, or try making a dish with simple, whole ingredients. These small steps can ignite a deeper transformation.

Chapter 3: The Down Fall of the Savage Life From a personal standpoint, I believe our modern diet of fast foods, hybridized, processed, ultraprocessed, toxified, genetically modified, nutrient-lacking foods, and our dietary habits attached to these packaged cardboard foods are misaligned with our evolutionary biology at the most basic of levels.

Many Americans are living longer than their parents, but they are not healthier, nor are they leading happier lives. When I ask my patients what their goals are, I learn just how hard they will work to get healthier. What many of them tell me is that "I do not want to live past 80", they perceive reaching this age is "old". They explain it to me, they do not want to be placed in a care facility, nor do they want to be cared for or dependent on their relatives.

What has happened to bring us to this point? Our Standard American Diet (SAD) has come to consist of mostly processed foods that are high in sugar and fat, and toxins. This diet emerged when agriculture began prioritizing yields and shelf-life over nutrition

Conventional and processed foods lack nutrient density, contributing to "hidden hunger" and has been at the forefront of the rise of chronic disease. In addition to lacking nutrition, industrial farming, directly and indirectly, affects human health via exposure to potentially toxic chemicals and environmental pollutants.

" Health is not just the absence of disease, and disease is not the absence of drugs."

Despite a clear connection between food and health, the current healthcare system in place in the United States underprioritizes nutrition education for medical students and diet-based nutrition plans. Our medical system is overburdened attempting to treat chronic disease with pharmaceutical interventions. It seems as if there is only one solution within our current medical care system; it offers only one solution, that is "A pill for an ill". Meanwhile, conventional farming systems rely on toxic inputs that degrade human health and prioritize crops low in nutritional value. With cancer rates and autoimmune diseases on the rise worldwide, and only 60 years of topsoil left due to soil degradation, we need a new path to improving human health. In 2014 Maria-Helena Semedo of the Food and Agriculture Organization warned that if current rates of soil degradation continued, all of the world's topsoil could be gone within 60 years.

Healthy soil is essential for nutrient-dense crops, yet we're losing it at an alarming rate—about 24 billion tons globally every year. Without urgent action, we risk depleting this resource entirely within 60 years.

There is new regenerative farming that is happening all around us by brave small farms. It is an approach that prioritizes the restoration and enhancement of soil health, including biodiversity and ecosystem functionality. Unlike conventional farming methods, which often deplete resources and degrade the environment over time, regenerative farming focuses on practices that rebuild soil fertility, sequester carbon in the soil, and promote resilience in agriculture systems.

Healthy soil increases water retention, nutrient availability and plant resilience. They incorporate diverse crops, and they cover crops which, when done during the off-season, it protects the soil from erosion, and enhances organic matter. When rotational grazing is practiced, it mimics natural ecosystems and supports biodiversity. They manage grazing cycles that mimic natural animal migration patterns, which promotes soil aeration, nutrient cycling, and grassland health. Healthy soil produces crops rich in vitamins, minerals, and antioxidants. When we deplete the soil, we deplete the food it grows—and, ultimately, ourselves.

There are many aspects of regenerative farming that the farmers of the past implemented simply because that was what worked. Not everything old is bad or outdated. I believe we need to either return to some of the practices we did before when it mattered to us, or we didn't eat. While industrial farming has wreaked havoc on human and environmental health, there is hope in the form of regenerative farming.

This approach not only restores the soil but also aligns with the sustainable practices our ancestors used

for millennia. Industrial farming relies on synthetic pesticides, herbicides, and fertilizers, which not only harm the soil but also leach into our water supply and food chain, contributing to hormone disruption, cancer, and other health issues.

" People are fed by the food industry, which pays no attention to health, and are treated by the health industry, which pays no attention to food." –Wendell Berry.

It has always baffled me on a very deep level, how the medical community can eat every day, and know that we as human beings have by and large eaten on a fairly frequent basis for at least 3 million years, and yet they always downplay the role of food and/or vitamins. Despite the clear link between food and health, medical schools devote an average of only 19 hours to nutrition education—less than 1% of their curriculum. This lack of training leaves doctors ill-equipped to address the root causes of diet-related diseases. It is especially disheartening to me when I think about the most basic of cycles within our body are all started with at least one vitamin, and at any given moment if you do not have enough of or have too much of a certain vitamin or element you can die. This is why certain vitamins and minerals are considered "essential". While all vitamins and minerals are considered essential for health, some deficiencies—such as Vitamin C, Vitamin B12, potassium, sodium, or iron—can quickly lead to lifethreatening conditions if not addressed. A balanced diet is crucial to avoid these critical deficiencies.

While we can't change the healthcare system overnight, we can take control of our own health by focusing on whole, nutrient-dense foods. Start by incorporating just one unprocessed, seasonal ingredient into your meals each day, and slowly build from there. By adopting even a fraction of Ekon's mindset, we can reclaim the vitality that modern life has stolen from us. Together, let's make choices that honor our bodies, respect the earth, and rebuild the connection we've lost—with food, nature, and ourselves.

The modern dietary challenges we face have become nearly overwhelming. Evidence that directly links our dietary habits and the food we eat to the impact on our health is emerging daily. Obesity now affects over 40% of American adults, and diabetes diagnoses have more than doubled in the past 20 years.

These trends are directly linked to the modern diet in straying from our evolutionary biology. Highly processed foods spike blood sugar, disrupt hormones, and create nutrient imbalances that drive chronic inflammation—a root cause of many modern diseases.

The story of Ekon reminds us that the wisdom of the past holds the key to a healthier, more vibrant future.

By embracing the principles of The Savage Diet, we can rediscover not only how to nourish our bodies, but how to live with purpose, gratitude, and harmony. The path forward is one of reconnection—with our food, our environment, and ourselves. Let's begin the journey together.

Section 1: A Savage Life

The early morning mist clung to the forest floor as Ekon crouched low, scanning for signs of life. The wind carried the sharp scent of pine as the sun broke over the horizon, casting long shadows across the open grassland. His companion Kirak stood close by, spear in hand, scanning the distant ridges for movement.

Behind Kirak, his two oldest children, Daro and Yema, stood ready to accompany Ekon this morning to help and learn. Their goal was clear: gather food to sustain the family and return before the sky turned gray with an approaching storm.

Ekon instructed them to follow the stream and collect tubers and roots. As they waded into the cold water, using their toes to grip the rocks, they would then stop to pick a tuber, and the thick cold mud would swallow their feet until they moved to the next tuber. They prodded the riverbank, each with a sharpened stick, loosening the soil to reveal thick starchy tubers, they did this until the sun was high in the sky. Kirak raised up to stretch his aching back when suddenly, he heard a small clinking in the nearby field. Looking up, and through the trees, he saw there was a small herd of elk present; their antlers were hitting one another as they grazed on the field of delicious grasses. He signaled Ekon, pointing to the

herd, and Ekon nodded, indicating he had also seen the elk. Ekon then gave a slight, quick movement of his hand to the children watching. They nodded their heads and both quietly exited the stream, crouching low behind a cluster of shrubs. A massive bull elk was grazing, standing near the edge of his herd, his antlers towering like a crown with its head dipping and rising as it nibbled at the undergrowth. Kirak steadied his breath, he raised his spear he had so painstakingly crafted with a stone tip tied securely to a wood shaft and let it fly with a swift, practiced motion. The weapon struck true, and as the elk fell heavily to the ground, he let out a guttural bellow, and the herd erupted into chaos. Startled by the sound and the sight of their fallen leader, the elk scattered in all directions, their hooves pounding the ground like thunder. Kirak and Ekon remained quiet, just watching the dust rise as the herd vanished into the forest.

The hunters slowly approached the elk, their senses were heightened. Watching warily to make sure there was no movement, to be sure that the elk was dead, was imperative, as the beast could rise suddenly and gore the unsuspecting hunter. They had seen this happen too many times not to be careful.

Kirak placed his hand on the chest of the elk, murmuring in their native tongue, "Thank you for your life".

Honoring the elk's spirit was imperative to ensure many more successful hunts. They then worked quickly, knowing that the fresh blood could attract predators. They skinned and prepared the meat, wrapping cuts in the elk hide for transport. The elk was so very large they needed to cut it up into large quadrants so that they could carry it out quickly. The sinew would be dried and twisted into sturdy cords for binding tools. The leg bones once hallowed and sharpened would serve as awls or needles for crafting hides into garments. The hide would become a new cloak or bed cover to keep warm through the winter. They needed to take all of the meat, or it would be scavenged by one of their daily predators, like a Sabor-toothed Tiger or the small-faced bear that would take over the carcass, and the hunters would lose their kill. Meanwhile, Daro and Yema had paused in their search for tubers while they quietly waited for Ekon and Kirak to bring down the elk. Now they went back to the creek, the season was getting colder, and they knew they could not stop in their search as the creek would be frozen solid soon and the tubers would be gone. Ekon returned to them and told them to continue to gather as much as they could carry; when their baskets were full, they were to return to the cave. He told them to look for the leaves with the deepest color as the good roots grow beneath these. As Ekon watched Daro and Yema by the creek, their small hands muddy from digging tubers, a sense of pride swelled within him. They were learning to provide, just as he had learned from his father. Yet, with winter's breath already in the air, a shadow of worry lingered. Would their efforts be enough to sustain the tribe through the harsh months ahead? There were several plants they would also pick to put into the gruel they would cook tonight.

Growing along the bank of the creek, there was mint and a tangle of small bitter berries. These would be dried by the fire and then they will sweeten and be a fine addition to the meal. Ekon and Kirak gathered all of the elk they could carry to head back to the cave, leaving the two young girls alone. Not long after Ekon and Kirak had left, the clouds began to gather overhead. Daro and Yema had stopped and were looking up at the sky, noting that their baskets were nearly full and heavy, so they came up out of the creek, their feet ice cold, they both began to shiver with the sudden wind and coldness of the air.

By the time the storm clouds rolled in, the family had reunited near their shelter of a cave with a rocky outcropping. To a stranger walking by, it would seem as if it was just a clump of rocks, but they had found a cave that was hidden from view in the rocks. It was dark at night, but as the dawn hit, it became lighter and warmer. The girls were just reaching the cave when Ekon came out. He and Kirak had gotten all of the meat out on the first trip so they would not need to go back. The girls were just as heavily laden with their burden of the tubers and various greens that they had gathered as they walked back to the cave.

He grabbed their heavy baskets and helped them place the tubers on the coals of the fire. They would let their skins blacken, and the insides soften, while the meat was placed on a spit roasting over the fire.

Mara, the girl's mother, spread the berries on a flat stone to dry. The greens were tossed in a clay pot with water to make a simple broth. The tubers' skins crackled as they blackened on the fire, releasing a smoky, sweet aroma that mingled with the rich scent of roasting meat. The broth simmered in the clay pot, flecks of green floating in the bubbling water. As the embers of the fire died down, they ate in silence, the crackling fire being the only sound. The venison was tender, the tubers sweet and smoky and as they

placed their hides around the fire that night, their bellies were full, and they were content. As the family drifted to sleep, their spirits were calm, they were at peace in a way that modern life has forgotten. In the simplicity of their day—the hunt, the gathering, the shared meal—they found connection, purpose, and contentment. These are the principles we must strive to reclaim.

In Ekon's world, every bite was earned through effort, patience, and connection to the land. There were no shortcuts, no processed foods to dull their senses or inflame their bodies. Their meals, though simple, were profoundly nourishing—a stark contrast to the empty calories and artificial ingredients found in the modern diet.

Section 2: The Beginning of the End

The modern diet, as we understand it today, is characterized by high intakes of processed foods, refined sugars, and industrial oils. This began to take shape during the Industrial Revolution, which started in the late 18th century and progressed throughout the 19th century. Where the main focus was on the mechanization of agriculture and textiles and it was also at this time that steam power became very important in moving industrialization to the next level. The second phase of industrialization saw the advancement of steel production, electricity, and then mass manufacturing. This period marked significant changes in food production, processing, and consumption patterns.

Here is a brief overview of how our modern diet has devolved into processed and genetically modified foods. Our diet has shifted from being genetically and evolutionarily sound to becoming the cause of disease within the humans it feeds. What happened? How did we go from nutrient-dense diets that supported human health for millennia to the processed, genetically modified foods that now dominate our plates? The answer lies in a series of transformations that began during the Industrial Revolution and continue to shape our diets today.

The Industrial Revolution brought mass production to food, mechanizing processes that had once been done by hand. During World War II, soldiers depended on canned rations—processed, shelf-stable meals designed for convenience, not nutrition. When the war ended, these foods found their way into civilian kitchens, changing the way we thought about eating. We saw the rise of canned foods and refined grain products, which could be produced in large quantities and stored for extended periods, facilitating urban supply and reducing seasonal food scarcity. The technologies such as canning, pasteurization, and later, refrigeration, were developed. These innovations extended food's shelf life but stripped away much of its nutritional value in the process.

We entered the era of monoculture farming. In other words, we eliminated the small farms across the United States. Monoculture farming—the repeated planting of the same crop—has devastated soil health, robbing it of the diverse nutrients that traditional farming once preserved. As a result, the food we grow today contains fewer vitamins and minerals than it did just a century ago. For example, a study showed that the iron content of spinach has decreased by nearly 50% since the 1950s. By prioritizing yield over quality, we've created a system that feeds more people but nourishes fewer. This shift was supported by synthetic fertilizers and pesticides, boosting yields but also beginning the decline in soil health and nutritional content of crops. Yes, that was not long ago. We then began introducing highyielding crop varieties, especially grains, which increased food availability, but often contained less protein and nutrients than traditional strains.

These shifts in farming and food production have had a profound impact on our health. The rise of processed and nutrient-deficient foods has been directly linked to skyrocketing rates of obesity, diabetes, heart disease, and autoimmune disorders. What began as a quest for convenience has turned into a global health crisis.

And yet again, we started the rise of convenience foods in the mid-1900s. After World War II, economic prosperity and the rise of consumer culture fueled an explosion of processed foods, from frozen dinners to sugary snacks. Convenience foods, including frozen meals, pre-packaged snacks, and fast food, have become popular and have not swayed in their overall popularity.

Then began the aggressive marketing campaigns promoting these new food products as symbols of modernity and convenience, significantly altering our dietary HABITS. Note the emphasis. Aggressive marketing campaigns didn't just sell food; they sold an idea. Convenience foods were positioned as symbols of progress, independence, and even luxury. By the 1950s, television ads showed happy families enjoying frozen dinners and sugary breakfast cereals, embedding processed foods into the fabric of American culture. Over time, this messaging eroded our ancestral relationship with food as nourishment, replacing it with a fixation on speed and ease.

Understanding how we arrived at this point is the first step in reclaiming our health. By recognizing the forces that shaped the modern diet, we can begin to unlearn harmful habits and reconnect with the wisdom of our ancestors. The Savage Diet offers a path forward—a way to align our eating habits with our biology and the natural rhythms of the earth.

Section 3: The Scientific History of Our Decline

The story of modern nutrition is one of good intentions gone wrong. From early observational studies to sweeping public health policies, the advice we've been given about what to eat has often been flawed—

and the consequences have been profound. To understand how we got here, we must first look at two men whose opposing ideas laid the foundation for our current dietary crisis: Weston A. Price and Ancel Keys.

Weston A. Price was a Canadian dentist who is best known for his theories on the relationship between nutrition, dental health, and physical health. Dr. Price initially started his career in dentistry in Cleveland, Ohio, where he was particularly interested in issues related to orthodontics and dental caries (cavities).

Dr. Price became increasingly concerned about the causes of dental problems among his patients, especially those related to tooth decay and facial deformities. This led him to undertake extensive research that focused on isolated human populations around the world. In the 1930s, he traveled to various parts of the world, including Africa, South America, North America, Australia, and the Polynesian islands, to study the diets and health of populations relatively untouched by Western civilization at that time. His observations and findings were compiled into his book "Nutrition and Physical Degeneration"

(1939), which is considered his seminal work. In this book, Dr. Price argued that many modern health problems were unheard of in non-Westernized societies, which he attributed to their consumption of traditional diets. He proposed something that was against what other people thought. He was thinking outside the box. He noted that these diets were rich in essential nutrients (particularly vitamins A and D, and what he termed "Activator X," now believed to be Vitamin K2) derived from animal fats, seafood, and other nutrient-dense foods. Dr. Price observed that the people he studied who consumed traditional diets had straight teeth, few cavities, and overall excellent dental health, whereas those who had adopted Westernized diets high in refined sugars and flours suffered from poor dental health and other health issues. Look at the teeth we have today. In the Swiss Alps, Price observed isolated communities thriving on diets of whole milk, cheese, and rye bread, with children displaying strong, straight teeth and robust health. In contrast, nearby villages that had adopted refined flour and sugar showed higher rates of cavities, crowded teeth, and illness.

While Price's work was pioneering at the time and remains influential in certain circles, particularly within the fields of holistic and alternative nutrition, it has been criticized for lacking rigorous scientific methodology. So, his conclusions about the superiority of traditional diets, while supported by detailed observations, often did not control for other variables that could affect health. Dr. Weston A. Price's research has had a lasting impact on nutritional theories, particularly influencing those who advocate for

whole food-based diets and those who oppose processed foods. His work helped to spur the modern movement that criticizes processed foods and underscores the potential health benefits of returning to more traditional, whole-food diets.

Price's observations remind us that the health of traditional populations wasn't an accident—it was the result of nutrient-dense, whole-food diets perfectly aligned with their environments. These principles form the backbone of The Savage Diet, proving that the wisdom of the past can guide us toward better health today.

The Weston A. Price Foundation, founded in 1999, continues to promote his ideas, advocating for the consumption of whole, traditionally prepared foods, and fats as a means to improve health and prevent disease. The foundation also critiques modern agricultural practices and supports organic and biodynamic farming methods.

I believe money has always been at the forefront of all of this, as everyone wanted to make a dime, but then it hit new levels. Starting with Ancel Keys.

Ancel Keys was an influential American scientist known for his research on dietary fats and their role in heart disease. One of his most famous studies, the Seven Countries Study, significantly shaped dietary guidelines in the United States and, sadly in other parts of the world. Keys' hypothesis became gospel, shaping the U.S. government's dietary guidelines and giving rise to the low-fat craze of the 1980s and 1990s. Food manufacturers replaced fats with refined carbohydrates and sugars, creating the 'fat-free'

products that dominated supermarket shelves—and unknowingly contributed to the obesity epidemic we face today.

However, the study and Keys' conclusions have been criticized for several methodological flaws and biases. Just not for many, many years. It was too late. The damage was done.

The Seven Countries Study, initiated in the late 1950s, examined the diets, lifestyles, and incidence of coronary heart disease in men from seven countries in different parts of the world (Italy, Greece, Yugoslavia, Finland, Netherlands, United States, and Japan).

Critics argue that Keys selectively included countries that supported his hypothesis, while excluding nations like France and Switzerland, where high saturated fat intake coincided with low rates of heart disease, as well as countries with low fat intake yet high rates of heart disease.

31

The study's design was observational and could only establish correlations rather than causation. While Keys highlighted the correlation between saturated fat intake and heart disease rates, this does not prove that one causes the other. There could be other contributing factors or confounders that were not controlled for in the study. The dietary complexity was ignored. The study primarily focused on the intake of saturated fats and its link to heart disease, largely ignoring other dietary components that could affect heart health, such as sugar, fiber, and overall diet quality. This was a one-size-fits-all approach. The conclusions drawn from the study led to broad dietary recommendations that did not account for individual variations in diet and lifestyle or genetic factors affecting heart disease.

The critics have accused Keys of cherry-picking data that supported his hypothesis while ignoring or dismissing data that did not. Some analyses may have been overly simplistic or inadequate to support the sweeping conclusions regarding the dangers of saturated fat. However, this influenced our policy on how and what to eat in the United States and was a major influence on the food pyramids, that we have all so faithfully followed throughout the years. Despite its flaws, the Seven Countries Study had a profound impact on demonizing saturated fats. This has been suggested to contribute to increased consumption of refined carbohydrates and sugars, aligning with rising obesity rates and metabolic syndromes globally.

In recent years, there has been a significant reevaluation of the data from the Seven Countries Study alongside newer research. This has led to a more nuanced understanding of fats, where the type of fat (such as the distinction between trans fats, saturated fats, and unsaturated fats) and the source of fat are considered important.

The role of dietary fats in heart disease remains a topic of ongoing research and debate, with more recent studies suggesting that the relationship between saturated fat and heart disease is not as clear-cut as once thought. Ancel Keys' work, while pioneering at the time, illustrates the complexities of nutritional science and the importance of rigorous methodology in research. His studies have prompted valuable discussions and further research into diet and heart disease, highlighting the need for continuous questioning and investigation in science.

And yet, we have two influential men, at slightly different times in the United States, expressing very clear subjective views. Dr. Price indicated through his exhaustive work and travels, that we need to go back to a more natural way of eating, avoiding sugars specifically and processed foods, although at that time, the number of processed foods was nearly insignificant as to how it is now. The amount of backlash and disregard for his findings, although subjective (with pictures) is noteworthy. Ancel Keys on the other hand, had just as subjective data, no pictures and he was believed outright. This, I believe, was the start of the decline of our health as we have known it. Scientifically, you have to look at it all, you cannot form an opinion until you do.

The removal of lard and animal fats from the diet, particularly in the mid-20th century, has had several unintended negative health consequences. While this shift was driven by efforts to reduce cardiovascular disease based on Ancel Keys' Seven Countries Study, subsequent research has revealed that replacing traditional animal fats with processed alternatives introduced its own set of health risks. When lard and animal fats were replaced with margarine and hydrogenated vegetable oils, trans fats entered our diets—

substances now linked to increased risks of heart disease, stroke, and type 2 diabetes. My patients tell me how their diets are. With few exceptions, they tell me they use vegetable oils, or if they do not knowingly use them, they go out and eat regularly. These are high in omega-6 fatty acids, e.g. soybean and corn oil and this is predominately what restaurants will use. This leads to excessive Omega-6

consumption relative to Omega-3s, which then promotes inflammation and is linked to chronic disease.

The takeaway is clear: we need to question conventional wisdom about nutrition and look to traditional diets for guidance. Avoiding processed oils, choosing whole animal fats, and incorporating nutrient-dense foods like grass-fed butter and organ meats can help restore the balance our bodies were designed for.

Part II: Mastering the Principles of The Savage Diet Chapter 4: Staying Committed to the Savage Diet

Section 1: The Power of Purpose

Why? The first step in committing to anything is understanding your Reason. Whether it's a relationship, a diet, or a way of coping with a diagnosis or a chronic illness, you must first ask yourself, why? This will be the motivation that keeps you going in whatever pursuit you choose. It will be the reason you get out of bed in the morning, and it all revolves around fulfilling that reason.

Write down your reasons and keep them handy, put them on your refrigerator, and visualize how you want to be. See the sleek body that you have wanted, or imagine your happiness in receiving an all-clear of a cancer diagnosis. Take 5 minutes each morning to visualize the person you want to become and how The Savage Diet aligns with that vision. This visualization will inspire you and remind you of the sense of achievement that comes with reaching your goals.

Celebrate with Milestones

Your environment plays a pivotal role in your success. A pantry stocked with nutrient-dense foods and free of inflammatory triggers (like processed snacks and seed oils) removes daily temptations. This supportive environment reassures you that you're not alone in your journey and that your surroundings are working with you, not against you.

Always attempt to declutter your kitchen and stock it with whole foods. Buy only grass-fed meats and fermented items. I recommend that you do as I did and invest in a great juicer, an Insta-pot and/or an air fryer, and a really good blender. For our busy lives, we need to do something to remove the angst.

Prepare your meals ahead of time and then either freeze or put the prepared meal in the refrigerator.

Sometimes, it is easier if you have your own tribe you can count on. If you surround yourself with people who share your values, or even an online support group it is easier to deal with the day-to-day problems that we encounter. You can share your story on www.thesavagediet.com.

Section 2: How to Navigate Parties and Social Gatherings

I recommend that you eat before you go to parties. Holidays and restaurant outings can be tricky, so if you eat before the event, you will not be starving and will not make less-than-ideal food choices. Plan ahead and bring a dish that aligns with your diet, it will be good simply because it has healthy items in it, it will have all of the spices and organic foods that people often wonder about but will be able to see and taste it.

Be strong and practice saying no to something that does not align with your dietary choices. Another option is also to opt for a simple meal - think grilled proteins and vegetables. The only possible problem with that is a question about the type of oils they may have used unless it is a grilled protein.

Section 3: What About Setbacks

I always recognize that my patients will fail at times. I try to foresee this and plan for it. I tell them I understand they will be placed in a position where they may make a choice not in keeping with their plan.

I understand. There is no need to beat yourself up and feel guilty, and there is nothing other than putting the resolve in your mind to be a little stronger next time and just say no. I find that this seems to make my patients feel better, and they move forward. I also have patients who for whatever reason, just cannot

move past their transgression, and they will stay in that mode of guilt. I do not judge at all. To me, there is no right or wrong in dealing with diet or healthy lifestyle choices. Consistency over time is more important than perfection. Everyone will get to the point where they feel great or have such improvements, it is only a matter of moving forward.

Practice Gratitude

Gratitude can shift your focus from what you are "missing" to what you are gaining. Take a moment daily or even twice a day to reflect on how your health, energy, or mood has improved since starting The Savage Diet.

Before you arise in the morning, take a few nice deep breaths, and then place your right hand over your heart, and close your eyes. Lay there, feeling the beat of your heart, feeling grateful for each beat.

Knowing that it can be just as easily be still and cold. My mother used to say to me "In the blink of an eye, go I". Be grateful for each and every moment. Make your plan for the day, and see yourself doing your plan. Be living in the moment.

Section 4: Harmonizing Home Life

Balancing home life while following The Savage Diet can be challenging, especially if you're juggling family responsibilities, work, and other obligations. However, with some thoughtful planning and flexibility, it can be integrated smoothly into your everyday routine. Here are some strategies to help balance home life while maintaining the principles of The Savage Diet

Try to plan and prepare your meals in advance. Spend a couple of hours each week preparing meals or meal components. You want to chop vegetables and marinate meats. It does not take that long, but just in case you want to spend more time preparing it is ok. I try to do batch cooking. For example, a large pot of stew or roasted meats and vegetables can be stored for several days, and then reassembled for your meals. You can adapt The Savage Diet principles to create family meals that everyone can enjoy.

Have the children help in preparing the food or the meals. Not only does this build responsibility, but they learn in the process.

If you have a family that has children, then I would recommend that you start with small changes. Swap out processed foods for whole-nutrient-dense options. Gradually shift everyone's eating habits without overwhelming yourself (and your family). Remember, if your children are eating a ton of carbohydrates and fast foods, or your spouse for that matter, then the challenge will be greater. If they are open to eating better and healthier, then great! Have a sit-down and talk out a plan. If they are not, then I always go to plan B. My plan is more psychological than anything, it works very well if you have a husband and a wife, but it will work with kids too; sometimes, it takes just a little longer.

Plan B: I take the willing participant, and help them, showing them what to do. I have never had anyone not be successful on The Savage Diet or The Savage Way of Life. The wife or husband that is willing just does the program, they will lose weight or gain weight, whatever is right for them. I tell them, not to say anything, just do the program. The other partner begins to see the changes and then begins to ask questions, and the rest as they say is history.

Section 5: Create a Consistent Routine

Set meal times by establishing regular meal times that work for your family and stick to them. This consistency will make it easier to incorporate The Savage Diet in your home life and prevent unhealthy snacking or last-minute pizza decisions. Make the whole week a time when the family must sit down and eat with one another. This is where the memories are made. Talk to your children and ask them questions about their day; really listen to them. Do not allow even one phone at the table. Place the

phones away from the table. Turn them off, it is ok, the world will still be spinning on its axis when the meal is finished, and you have not looked at your phone even once. I remember all of the years when there were no phones at all, except the one in the kitchen with a long cord attached to it. Trust me, you will thank me when your kids are older, and years from now they will talk and laugh about some of the things said at the table.

Prepare your snacks

Have things like precut fruits and vegetables, homemade energy bars or nuts ready when you need something quick.

Stay Flexible

Be adaptable. Life at home does not always go according to plan, and sometimes, you may need to adjust the diet to fit your circumstances. If you are having a busy day, opt for simpler meals or choose leftovers. If you have social events or family gatherings, make adjustments without feeling guilty – focus on your goals in the long term.

Balance Meal Diversity and Simplicity

Not every meal needs to be a complex recipe. Many aspects of The Savage Diet can be simplified, such as focusing on protein (e.g., eggs, meat) and vegetables, or preparing simple salads with a protein topping. Having easy-to-make meals will reduce the stress of sticking to the diet.

Chapter 5 - Your Savage Journey

Section 1: In the Shadow of Time

Beneath the ancient amber sky,

Where glaciers loomed and winds would sigh,

The hunter stalked with silent tread,

Through whispers where the wild ones fed.

A spear of stone, a heart of steel,

Each step a prayer, each breath concealed. The

earth, his map, the trail his guide,

Through shadows deep, where secrets bide.

The beast, majestic, grazed alone,

Its frame a fortress, muscle and bone. Unaware

of eyes that bore,

The hunger of the tribesmen's lore.

With wind aligned and patience honed,

The hunter crouched, his aim enthroned. A

moment stretched, the stillness deep, The

world inhaled, the land asleep.

The spear flew swift, its arc a song,

A melody of right and wrong. It

struck its mark; the beast did cry,

An echo torn from earth to sky.

In death, there lived a sacred rite, Of life

exchanged beneath the night. The

hunter bowed, his thanks bestowed, For

what the spirits had bestowed.

And so, beneath the starlit dome,

He bore the gift of life back home. A

tale of courage, fire, and strife,

Etched forever in the hunt of life.

"Every journey begins with a single step, but the Savage Journey
begins with a choice: the decision to reclaim your health, strength,
and vitality." The hunter's journey in the poem is not so different
from your own. Every step he takes, every breath he draws, is part
of a greater rhythm—the rhythm of survival, resilience, and
connection to the earth. Like the hunter, your Savage Journey
begins with awareness and a willingness to embrace the challenges
ahead. It is a journey of courage, patience, and transformation.

In the hunter's world, survival depended on his ability to align with the natural rhythms of the earth—the wind, the sun, the seasons. Your Savage Journey is no different. By tuning into the rhythms of your body, reconnecting with the food and movement that nourished our ancestors, and honoring the cycles of rest and renewal, you can rediscover the vitality that has always been within you.

This is where the rubber meets the road—the moment where you step into your power and begin your journey of transformation. To discover yourself and all that you can do. I believe in you and I know that you will do the very best that you can.

The Savage Journey is not just about food, it is a holistic journey and transformation of your body, of your mind, and of the spirit within you. This might begin with something as simple as swapping out a processed snack for a handful of nuts or walking barefoot on the grass to reconnect with the earth. Over time, these small changes build into profound transformations: the energy you thought was gone returns, your body sheds what no longer serves it, and your mind becomes clearer and more focused. Each step, no matter how small, brings you closer to the vibrant health you deserve.

I know how frustrating it can be to feel like you've tried everything—only to watch the weight creep back on, or to wake up each morning feeling just as tired as the day before. These struggles aren't failures; they're signs that your body is crying out for change. And the good news is, that change is possible. You have the power to rewrite your story, one step at a time. I understand you may be struggling with health issues, possibly a lack of energy, daily. If you have a diagnosed health condition like diabetes or heart disease, or your doctor is saying you need to go on a statin drug, and you do not want to do this, but you do not know where to turn, I ask that you turn the page, take one more step. You can turn your health around, but you have to commit and take one more step, every day. Over time, these small changes build into profound transformations: the energy you thought was gone returns, your body sheds what no longer serves it, and your mind becomes clearer and more focused. Each step, no matter how small, brings you closer to the vibrant health you deserve."

Section 2: Awakening Your Awareness

I want you to sit down and reflect on your current health habits. What do you do on a daily basis to maintain or keep your health? Start journaling on your dietary habits and your emotions around foods.

Journal about what you did today—whether it's a 20-minute walk, choosing a healthier meal, or simply drinking more water. Celebrate your progress each week, like increasing your walk to 30 minutes or noticing how much better you feel. Keep your journal and you will see in one month how you have improved.

Your journal can become a powerful tool for self-awareness and growth. Here are some prompts to guide you:

•

What did I eat today, and how did it make me feel?

•

Did I move my body today? How did I feel before and after?

-

What emotions did I notice today, and how might they have influenced my food choices?

-

What is one small step I can take tomorrow to improve my health?

Journaling is about more than just tracking your habits—it's about reconnecting with yourself and your body's natural rhythms. In The Savage Diet, awareness is the first step to reclaiming the intuitive wisdom our ancestors lived by. By reflecting on your choices and how they make you feel, you'll begin to align your habits with what truly nourishes you—physically, mentally, and emotionally.

I recommend that you visit your physician first and get their okay to embark on a walking program or sit in the chair and do chair aerobics. If it has been some time since you had blood work done, get that done and have them explain it to you. When I review blood work with my patients, I ensure they leave with a clear understanding of their current health—and, more importantly, the steps they need to take to improve it. If there is a gut test we need to do based on their history, then we will do that. Healing your gut is one of the most powerful steps you can take to restore your health. By addressing the damage caused by years of poor dietary habits, you'll strengthen your immune system and reduce symptoms like joint pain and fatigue. It is usually joint pain, I find when I start healing the gut, the joint pain dissipates. The cleaner the diet, the healthier you become.

Your gut is often referred to as your 'second brain' because it plays a crucial role in regulating your immune system, mood, and overall health. When your gut is out of balance—due to processed foods, stress, or inflammation—it can lead to symptoms like joint pain, fatigue, and digestive discomfort. By prioritizing a diet rich in whole, unprocessed foods and reducing inflammatory triggers, you can begin to restore balance in your gut and experience significant improvements in your health.

Start with small changes that can make a big impact on your gut health. Incorporate foods like fermented vegetables, plain yogurt, or bone broth into your meals, and aim to eat a variety of fiber-rich vegetables to support a diverse microbiome. Even small adjustments, like drinking more water or taking a 10-minute walk after meals, can help your body begin to heal.

When you visit your physician, ask for a comprehensive blood panel that includes markers like CRP

(Creactive protein) for inflammation, Vitamin D levels, and fasting glucose. These tests can provide valuable insights into your current health and help guide the changes you need to make.

Section 3: Adopting the Savage Principles

Imagine a diet that not only fuels your body but heals it—a way of eating that aligns with your biology and connects you to the wisdom of the past. Adopting the principles of The Savage Diet means saying goodbye to processed, convenience-driven foods and embracing the natural, nutrient-rich foods our bodies were designed to thrive on. This is your path to strength, vitality, and balance."

Embracing whole, nutrient-dense foods involves shifting your focus from processed, convenience-driven eating to consuming foods that are as close to their natural state as possible. This change is about nourishing your body with essential nutrients while honoring the primal roots of human health. I am not asking you to go out and start hunting down your meat. I am asking you to choose wisely when you go to the grocery store.

First of all, focus on shopping the outer edges of the grocery store, where you'll find fresh, whole foods like produce, meats, and dairy. The center aisles are dominated by highly processed products. Choose organic grass-fed meats and organic pasture-raised eggs. Choose fresh vegetables, especially the leafy greens, all colors of the rainbow for fruit and vegetables, nuts and seeds. While there are things that can be omitted on the label, when they say organic and grass-fed, it is likely true. If anything has a bar-code, then I would use an app like YUKA to ensure there are no additional ingredients that would not be in your best interest to eat. For example, if you choose to buy a pancake batter, check the ingredients to make sure that it does not have ingredients that can harm your kidneys or disrupt your bone health. The YUKA app is great for this, you can see at a glance if the food has any ingredients that are harmful.

Choose natural, nutrient-dense fats like grass-fed, organic butter, ghee, lard, tallow, coconut oil, and extra virgin olive oil to support your body and reduce inflammation.

As we move forward with outlining the diet, I would invite you to avoid any empty calories, which would be processed foods, as they are high in calories, but low in nutrients, which will contribute to deficiencies and weight-gain.

If you are afraid to start on a whole food, nutrient-dense way of eating, then start with one day, juice a smoothy. Drink that one thing down, add more vegetables than fruit, and do this the first week. Or, if you prefer, you can juice with a juicer, start with that for one week, and then you will be ready to incorporate meals into your daily events.

Legumes are a food that has been used for thousands of years, but not so much during our time frame of The Savage Diet. Legumes are beans, lentils, chickpeas, and peas among others. As hunter-gatherers we did not consume them, it was more common when we became farmers and were a part of the

agricultural society that we started developing and consuming them. I believe that our hunter-gatherer society understood they contain phytates and lectins which are considered anti-nutrients because they can inhibit the absorption of minerals or irritate the gut in many people. The proper cooking techniques would not have been widely available to our Savage people, although they may have done so.

If you want to choose a small simple way to swap out changes, you can do sourdough bread instead of white bread. Swap out your vegetable oils for butter, ghee, or Extra Virgin olive oil and choose fresh fruits, nuts, or seeds instead of a sugary snack. Prioritize quality over quantity. Focus on a singleingredient food, e.g. a carrot vs a packaged "veggie snack". Go to your local farmers market, go to your local health food grocery store. Make your plate of fresh, non-starchy vegetables like spinach, kale, broccoli or bell peppers. Use fresh herbs and spices to enhance the flavor instead of relying on processed dressings.

Rotate between different sources of foods. For example, use beef and lamb and always choose organic, grass-fed cuts. Use wild-caught salmon, sardines, and mackerel for Omega-3s. Pasture-raised eggs are natural powerhouses and easy to find anywhere in your neighborhood. Some people have trouble eating organ meats, but they are exceptional nutrient rich foods. Out of all of the people I know, there is only one person who eats liver and onions, but he does so and loves it. I remember growing up, my Dad ate liver and onions a couple of times a month and although he had me taste it, at the time, I didn't really like the taste, but I encourage everyone to try it, at least once.

Ditch your industrial seed oils and start using fats like grass-fed butter and ghee. I use Extra-Virgin Olive oil for salads, and I always use bacon grease or coconut oil for cooking. I prepare meals like soups, stews or roasted vegetables in bulk, and I keep it simple and as straightforward as possible. An example of a typical meal for me would be grilled tri-tip (grass-fed and organic of course), organic steamed veggies, and an organic avocado on a bed of organic baby greens, with a medley of spices to create different flavors.

Industrial seed oils, such as soybean, corn, and canola oils, are highly processed and oxidize easily, leading to inflammation in the body. Our ancestors relied on natural fats like animal fats and olive oil, which are stable and rich in nutrients. By returning to these traditional fats, you can reduce inflammation and promote better overall health. I have patients ask me constantly about Avocado oil. It has been my experience, and while it seems like it is a healthy oil, remember that it has to be extracted from the seed.

It is a seed oil, and this usually means that they have to put it under pressure, and infuse Hexane into it to extract the oil. There are very few Avocado oils that I would consider safe to use, because of the extraction method. However, to eat an avocado, is just fine.

My rule is simple: if a product has more than four ingredients, or if the ingredients include names I can't pronounce, I leave it on the shelf. It just is not worth it to me. I use the YUKA app which makes shopping so much easier, especially when I am looking to buy something with a bar code. Every bite of food is a choice— one that can bring you closer to vibrant health or further from it. By choosing whole, nutrientdense foods, you're not just nourishing your body; you're honoring the wisdom of our ancestors and investing in a future where you feel energized, strong, and alive.

Batch cooking can save you time and ensure you always have healthy options on hand. Roast a large tray of mixed vegetables, prepare a pot of bone broth for soups, and grill several portions of grass-fed meat at once. Store these in glass containers so you can mix and match throughout the week for quick, nutrient-dense meals.

So, for all of this trouble, what will you get? My experience has shown me that one of the first things that happens is that you will experience more energy without any crashing. There will also be improved digestion; the high fiber and enzyme content in whole foods supports gut health. If you do not feel better,

then go to your doctor and get some blood tests done. Your immunity will improve, and as such, your skin will be clearer. You should also notice that your mood improves.

Chapter 6: Unlocking Nutrient Potential: Mastering Advanced Bioavailability The air was still cool from the night as Ekon stepped out of the rock shelter where his family slept. The sky was streaked with the first hint of dawn, and the scent of the damp earth filled his lungs. Today, would be like so many days before, survival would mean moving forward – seeking the food and resources that the land provided. The thought of what lay ahead was daunting, but he felt the steady rhythm of purpose beating within him.

The families of their small group would start today, and would travel for many days, following the river that cut through the valley as a silvery guide. The older hunters spoke of a grazing ground farther downriver, where herds of red deer and an ancient cattle species called "aurochs" were located. These cattle species were very large and so the promise of an abundant game was the group's motivation, but the journey required more than hope. Every step demanded vigilance; watching for signs of predators, listening for the telltale movement in the underbrush, and scanning the horizon for signs of smoke or rival tribes. Ekons stomach growled as he set out to gather early morning sustenance for everyone. He moved slowly and deliberately, bending to pluck leaves from a patch of wild greens he recognized from his mother's teachings. Not far away, he spotted the deep colored blossoms of tuber-bearing plants.

Using a simple digging stick that he fashioned from a sturdy branch, he unearthed a small bounty of roots. These would sustain the children and the elders while the hunters pursued larger game. By midmorning the group had stopped at a small meadow, there were a number of hoofprints here, pressed into the soft earth, heading towards a larger nearby meadow. While the hunters were getting their spears ready and doing last-minute repairs to make sure the spear would be true, the elders walked with the children, sharing the tales of past migrations and lessons learned along the way. For Ekon, these stories were powerful tales of survivability. He had learned much from these very same stories that had been passed down to him in the same way as was being done for these children.

As the sun reached its zenith, the group paused to rest under the shade of trees near the riverbank. The adults began to prepare a midday meal of the roots that they had gathered as they walked, they also had dried fish from the stream that they prepared to share with everyone. That evening the hunter's efforts bore fruit. A single deer, was felled with precision and care, providing enough meat to last for several days. They all sat and ate around the fire, singing and giving thanks to their holy one. They ate sparingly, ensuring there would be enough to smoke and preserve for the days ahead.

Tactics on The Savage Diet involve optimizing nutrient intake, enhancing bioavailability, and tailoring dietary practices to achieve specific health, performance, and longevity goals. These tactics take The Savage Diet principles further, ensuring maximum benefit from nutrient-dense, ancestral foods while addressing modern needs.

Ekon's journey reminds us of a truth that has endured through the ages: survival and vitality are built on the foundation of resourceful choices and a deep respect for food. While our lives today may not involve the same physical demands, the principles of ancestral eating still hold the key to unlocking our optimal health. In the modern world, we have the tools and knowledge to refine these principles into advanced tactics that meet our unique needs.

Section 1: Advanced Nutritional Tactics

Advanced nutritional tactics are about refining your diet to achieve the greatest possible benefit from nutrient-dense, ancestral foods. This means focusing on three key areas:

1. Optimizing Nutrient Intake – Choosing foods and preparation methods that maximize bioavailability.

2. Enhancing Digestive Health – Healing the gut to better absorb nutrients.

3. Tailoring Practices for Your Goals – Incorporating strategies like intermittent fasting, cyclical eating, and targeted supplementation to support energy, performance, and longevity.

Fermented foods like sauerkraut, kimchi, and kefir are rich in probiotics, which support gut health and enhance nutrient absorption. Fermentation also breaks down anti-nutrients like phytates, making minerals like iron and zinc more bioavailable. Incorporating even small amounts of fermented foods into your meals can have a profound impact on digestion and overall health.

Bone broth is a nutrient powerhouse, rich in collagen, gelatin, and amino acids that support joint health, gut lining repair, and skin elasticity. Simmering bones with a splash of vinegar for 12-24 hours extracts these nutrients, making broth an essential addition to your Savage routine.

Cyclical eating—alternating periods of nutrient-dense eating with short fasting windows—can help regulate hormones, improve insulin sensitivity, and enhance cellular repair. For example, try fasting for 12-16 hours overnight and focusing on high-quality fats, proteins, and vegetables during your eating window.

While organ meats like liver, heart, and kidneys may be an acquired taste, they are among the most nutrient-dense foods available. Packed with Vitamins A, B12, and minerals like iron and copper, these ancestral superfoods provide nutrients in their most bioavailable forms. Start by adding small amounts to ground meats or experimenting with recipes that balance their flavor.

For athletes or those with active lifestyles, focus on incorporating protein-rich foods like organic grass-fed beef and wild-caught fish to support muscle repair. If you're managing a chronic condition like diabetes, prioritize low-glycemic vegetables and healthy fats to stabilize blood sugar. For longevity, consider adding antioxidant-rich foods like berries, herbs, and spices to combat oxidative stress.

How you prepare your food matters just as much as what you eat. Soaking and sprouting grains, seeds, and legumes reduces anti-nutrients like lectins and phytates, making minerals like magnesium and zinc easier to absorb. Slow cooking methods like roasting and braising preserve nutrients while enhancing flavor, making meals more satisfying and nourishing.

Ekon's tribe survived through resourcefulness, determination, and respect for the land's bounty. In today's world, you have the opportunity to take these principles even further. By adopting advanced nutritional tactics, you can fine-tune your diet to support your unique health goals. Start small—try a new preparation method, add fermented foods to your meals, or experiment with fasting. Each step brings you closer to living in harmony with your body and rediscovering the vitality you were born to have.

Section 2 – Optimizing Nutrient Bioavailability

When your body can't absorb nutrients effectively, even the healthiest diet can leave you feeling tired, inflamed, or nutrient-deficient. For example, if your gut struggles to absorb calcium, you may experience weaker bones over time. Similarly, poor iron absorption can lead to anemia, fatigue, and difficulty focusing. By optimizing bioavailability, you ensure your body gets the full benefit of the nutrients you consume, supporting better energy, immunity, and overall health."

Optimizing nutrient bioavailability involves ensuring that your body effectively absorbs and utilizes the nutrients from your diet, making every bite count. Most people do not consider the proportion of nutrients that enter their bloodstream and what, if anything, is actually used by the body. Bioavailability also pertains to what occurs after digestion. If your gut struggles to digest food properly or your short-chain

fatty acids are imbalanced, your body cannot absorb the nutrients it requires to function optimally. This imbalance can affect your overall health and complicate weight loss. In my experience, if the gut is not balanced, it significantly hinders a person's ability to lose weight. While it is not the only factor, if the body is unbalanced, it becomes very challenging to lose weight. An imbalanced gut affects weight loss in multiple ways. First, poor nutrient absorption can lead to cravings and overeating as your body seeks the nutrients it's missing. Second, inflammation caused by gut imbalances can disrupt hormone signaling, including insulin and leptin, which regulate hunger and fat storage. Finally, a damaged gut lining can interfere with energy production, making it harder to stay active and burn calories. By restoring gut balance, you create the conditions for sustainable weight loss.

Certain nutrients are better absorbed when paired together. For instance, pairing iron-rich foods like spinach with Vitamin C sources like citrus fruits enhances iron absorption. Similarly, eating fat-soluble vitamins (A, D, E, and K) with healthy fats like avocado or olive oil ensures your body can use them effectively.

Foods like legumes, nuts, and grains contain anti-nutrients like phytates and lectins that can block nutrient absorption. Soaking, sprouting, or fermenting these foods helps reduce anti-nutrient content, making minerals like zinc and magnesium more available to your body.

A healthy gut is critical for nutrient absorption. Incorporating fermented foods like sauerkraut, kimchi, and kefir can help restore gut balance. Probiotic supplements and prebiotic fibers from foods like garlic, onions, and asparagus also promote a thriving microbiome.

Avoid processed foods. These foods not only lack nutrients but can also interfere with nutrient absorption.

For instance, high sugar intake can disrupt the gut microbiome, and synthetic additives may burden the digestive system.

Replacing processed foods with whole, natural options is a crucial step in enhancing bioavailability.

Optimizing your nutrient bioavailability isn't just about choosing the right foods—it's about helping your body unlock the full potential of those nutrients. Begin by adding one new habit this week, whether it's pairing foods strategically, soaking grains, or incorporating more fermented foods. Small changes can lead to big results, and your body will thank you for it.

Section 3: Short Chain Fatty Acids

Short-chain fatty acids (SCFAs) such as butyrate, acetate, and propionate are generated when beneficial gut bacteria ferment dietary fiber. These compounds play a critical role in gut health by strengthening the gut lining, reducing inflammation, and improving nutrient absorption. To boost SCFA production, focus on fiber-rich foods such as leafy greens, flaxseeds, and root vegetables.

There are a few Short Chain Fatty Acids (SCFA) that I deal with daily. I speak to my patients about the Gut sample they submitted, and I have found few people who are balanced, well I have not found anyone with a balanced microbiome. The key type of SCFAs is Acetate, which is the most abundant. The body uses this as an energy source and additionally, it is also involved in fat metabolism.

The next SCFA is Propionate, which supports glucose production and energy regulation. It also possesses some anti-inflammatory properties. The third type of SCFA is Butyrate, which is the most popular SCFA and has gotten a lot of free press on the internet. This is the primary energy source for the colon cells and it is critical for maintaining the gut barrier integrity and reducing inflammation. Butyrate is the main energy source for the cells that line your colon, helping to keep your gut barrier strong and healthy. This strengthens your immune system and reduces inflammation linked to conditions like IBS and

Crohn's disease. All of the SCFA acids strengthen the intestinal lining, which in turn helps prevent a

"leaky gut". Additionally, the SCFAs stimulate the release of hormones like GLP-1 and PYY, which promote satiety and reduces the appetite.

There are studies that indicate Butyrate in particular has demonstrated significant anti-cancer effects, particularly in colorectal cancer. Specifically inhibiting the proliferation of colon cancer cells in a cell typespecific and apoptosis-dependant manner in colon cancer cells, while supporting healthy cells. Oncel S, Safratowich BD, Lindlauf JE, et al. Nutrients. 2024;16(4):529. doi:10.3390/nu16040529.

So how do we get SCFAs? They are created when gut bacteria break down fermentable fiber, also known as prebiotics, that humans cannot digest. SCFAs can be recovered in the systemic circulation, where they play roles in glucose and lipid metabolism, as well as immune function. The foods that are high in fermentable fibers include fruits, vegetables, legumes, whole grains, and nuts. You can boost SCFA production by eating resistant starches, such as green bananas, cold rice, or chilled potatoes, which feed beneficial gut bacteria. Eating what you need is the best, if you do not have intestinal permeability and not knowing what foods you may have sensitivities to. I encourage everyone to have their gut microbiome evaluated with testing, to see where you are, and also to see what you need to do to become healthier.

Fusco W, Lorenzo MB, Cintoni M, et al. Nutrients. 2023;15(9):2211. doi:10.3390/nu15092211.

There are two bacteria Phyla of Bacteroidetes and Firmicutes digest these fibers through fermentation, releasing the SCFA as byproducts. I tell people on a daily basis, that balance in your gut is best. The Firmicutes are primarily Gram-positive bacteria and include Genera such as Clostridium, Lactobacillus and Bacillus. They are known for their ability to ferment dietary fibers into SCFAs like Butyrate and are crucial for maintaining gut health and epithelial integrity. Firmicutes has also been associated with various health conditions, including obesity, and metabolic disorders, especially where the Firmicutes/Bacteroidetes ratio is noted to be in an imbalanced state.

The balance between Firmicutes and Bacteroidetes—two major groups of gut bacteria—is critical for maintaining health. Firmicutes are known for producing SCFAs like butyrate, which support gut and metabolic health. However, an overabundance of Firmicutes compared to Bacteroidetes has been linked to obesity and metabolic issues. Striking the right balance supports healthy weight regulation and overall gut health.

Bacteroides on the other hand is a Gram-negative bacteria. This bacterium is adept at breaking down complex polysaccharides, including those found in the diet, but also those in the body mucosal layer, into simpler molecules that can be utilized by the host and other gut microbes. Bacteroidetes are also known for their role in maintaining gut homeostasis and preventing colonization by pathogenic bacteria. I have performed >800 tests that evaluate this gut microbiome, most people also come with the complaint that they can't seem to lose weight. I have not yet seen one person that the Firmicutes and Bacteroidetes were in balance. The gut matters. Sun Y, Zhang S, Nie Q, et al How SCFAs Compare to Other Fatty Acids

Short-Chain Fatty Acids

Medium-Chain Fatty Acids

Long-Chain Fatty Acids

Aspect

(SCFAs)

(MCFAs)

(LCFAs)

Length

2–5

6–12

13+

(Carbons)

Source

Fermentation of dietary fiber Coconut oil, palm kernel oil

Animal fats, vegetable oils

Energy storage and cell

Primary Role Gut and metabolic health

Rapid energy source

structure

Absorbed via lymphatic

Absorption

Produced in the colon

Directly absorbed in the liver system

So how do you keep your gut in a balanced state? One of the easiest and oldest ways to do this is to ferment your food, or if that is not possible, then eat fermented foods. If you ferment vegetables like sauerkraut and kimchi, this will enhance gut health by increasing probiotics and reducing all anti-nutrients.

You can also use fermented daily by drinking kefir and yogurt, these will improve lactose digestibility and provide beneficial bacteria. You can also combine Vitamin C-rich foods (e.g. citrus fruits, bell peppers) with non-heme sources, (e.g. spinach and beans) to enhance iron absorption (Cook & Monson, 1977).

With the fat-soluble vitamins; Vitamins A, D, E and K require dietary fat for absorption (Borelet et al., 2013).

We soak and sprout our seeds and nuts to reduce the phytic acid, to enhance nutrient absorption and make them easier to digest. You can lightly steam or blanch certain vegetables, like kale or spinach to reduce oxalates while it retains the nutrients. When we want bone broth, we slow cook them, as the bones release minerals like calcium, magnesium, and collagen, which supports joint health and gut integrity. Think of your gut microbiome as a bustling community where SCFAs act as fuel for the system.

Fiber-rich foods are like fertilizer for the 'good bacteria,' helping them produce SCFAs that strengthen your gut lining and protect your overall health.

Eat a diet that includes fibers, mostly consisting of plant-based foods to support diverse gut bacteria. Try to include resistant starches like cooled potatoes or reheated rice. This goes without saying; minimize or better yet, do not include any processed foods in your diet at all. All sugars and refined carbohydrates disrupt the gut microbiome, so limit that for sure.

Side Note: One of my patients, a mother of three, came to me frustrated by her inability to lose weight despite eating a 'healthy' diet. After testing her gut microbiome, we discovered an imbalance between her Firmicutes and Bacteroidetes, and she had very low SCFA production. By adding more fiber-rich foods, resistant starches like cold potatoes, and fermented foods to her diet, she not only lost 15 pounds over three months but also noticed improved energy and digestion.

Your gut health is the foundation of your overall well-being, and SCFAs are the key to unlocking its potential. Start by adding fiber-rich foods like leafy greens and root vegetables to your meals, experimenting with fermented foods like sauerkraut, or trying resistant starches like cooled potatoes.

Small changes can have a big impact—your gut, and your body, will thank you.

Section 4: Nutrient Cycling

Imagine it's winter, 20,000 years ago. The land is frozen, and fruits and vegetables are nowhere to be found. Instead, you rely on dried meat, animal fat, and marrow to sustain you. Fast forward to summer, when the earth blooms with leafy greens, wild berries, and roots. This natural ebb and flow of foods shaped our ancestors' health and metabolic flexibility—an instinctive form of nutrient cycling. Today, we can harness these same principles to optimize our health, no matter the season.

This is introducing different cycles of eating, ensuring a balance of nutrients and metabolic flexibility. It is touted as preventing nutrient imbalances and food sensitivities. It improves your metabolic flexibility and insulin sensitivity, which encourages fat loss. Introducing nutrient cycling is a choice. So, what does that have to do with The Savage Diet? I believe that our ancestors unknowingly did Nutrient cycling. For example, in spring and summer, fruits, leafy greens, and roots were abundant, providing a natural source of carbohydrates and vitamins.

In the fall the nuts and tubers would have been harvested and stored, and in the winter the more animalbased foods, dried meat and fats became the primary sources of nutrition. This created a natural variation in macronutrient and micronutrient intake over the course of time. Our ancestors were opportunistic in their eating habits, in other words they ate what they could find or hunt which led to periods of nutrient abundance and of course scarcity. The diet that we had was diverse as it was rich in

fibers, which promoted a healthy microbiome, which in turn helped produce short-chain fatty acids enhancing the nutrients to be absorbed.

Nutrient cycling isn't just about variety—it's a powerful tool for addressing modern health concerns. For instance, alternating macronutrients can improve insulin sensitivity, making it easier for your body to regulate blood sugar and burn fat. Calorie cycling can help you avoid metabolic slowdowns that often occur with prolonged dieting. Together, these techniques enhance metabolic flexibility, allowing your body to adapt to changing energy needs and avoid storing excess fat.

There are several different types of nutrient cycling that I will outline for you to possibly consider. To me this is to stimulate autophagy (cellular cleaning) and enhances longevity. Autophagy is your body's natural

'cellular cleaning' process, where old or damaged cells are broken down and recycled. Nutrient cycling can help stimulate this process, promoting longevity and overall health.

One type of nutrient cycling is called Macronutrient cycling, which involves varying the proportions of proteins, fats and carbohydrates in your diet over days or weeks. In the chart below you will see how this differentiates between 20,000 years ago and what we could do today.

Alternate between high-protein, low-carb days (to promote fat burning) and high-carb, moderate-protein days (to fuel activity and replenish glycogen stores).

Comparison of Macronutrient Patterns

Aspect

Diet 20,000 Years Ago

Modern Nutrient Cycling

High after a hunt, low during lean

High-protein days alternate with low-protein

Protein Intake

times.

days.

Carbohydrate

Seasonal: Higher in summer/fall (fruits,

Intake

Intentional carb cycling for energy or fat loss.

roots).

High during winter (animal fat,

Alternates based on goals (ketogenic periods

Fat Intake

marrow).

or moderate fat).

Feast and famine cycles based on

Calorie cycling to match energy expenditure

Calorie Intake

food availability.

or fat loss goals.

Micronutrient variability can also be planned by rotating foods rich in specific vitamins and minerals (e.g., alternating magnesium-rich greens and zinc-rich seeds).

Key Differences

Aspect

Ancient Diet

Modern Nutrient Cycling

Dependent on environmental

Control

Fully controlled and tailored by the individual.

conditions.

Limited by geography and

Variety

Unlimited access to diverse foods year-round.

seasons.

Purpose

Survival and sustenance.

Health optimization, performance, and aesthetics.

Nutrient

Wild foods rich in nutrients.

Modern foods vary; nutrient density depends on choices

Density

(e.g., organic, unprocessed).

Micronutrient Rotation

Rotate foods rich in specific nutrients, such as zinc (pumpkin seeds, shellfish) one day and magnesium (dark leafy greens, nuts) the next. This ensures a broad spectrum of vitamins and minerals.

Seasonal Eating

Focus on foods naturally available in each season—leafy greens and berries in summer, root vegetables and squashes in fall, and fattier meats in winter.

Calorie Cycling

Plan lower-calorie days during rest periods and higher-calorie days when you're active or recovering from intense exercise.

Nutrient cycling invites you to embrace the natural rhythms of eating that sustained our ancestors for millennia. Whether you start with a simple seasonal approach or experiment with macronutrient cycling, every step brings you closer to metabolic balance, greater energy, and improved health. Listen to your body, make small changes, and let your instincts guide you—it's time to rediscover the art of eating in harmony with nature.

Section 5: The Benefits of Emulating Ancient Patterns

Nutrient cycling in modern diets can replicate some of the benefits our ancestors enjoyed in their eating patterns. They had metabolic flexibility, although they probably did not realize it but cycling between highcarb and low-carb days would mimic periods of feasting on seasonal fruits and fasting. Their gut health would have been robust because of their diverse plant-based foods. The periodic calorie cycling and fasting would have promoted hormone regulation.

Metabolic flexibility allows your body to switch seamlessly between burning carbohydrates and fat for energy, which promotes sustained energy levels and reduces the risk of metabolic disorders like insulin resistance. Our ancestors naturally developed this ability through alternating periods of feast and scarcity.

Similarly, their diverse plant-based diets supported a healthy gut microbiome, which we know is essential for digestion, immunity, and even mood regulation.

For example, our ancestors might feast on wild berries and roots in the summer, providing their bodies with a high-carb boost. In contrast, winter months would shift their diet to fat-rich animal foods, naturally mimicking the effects of a low-carb or ketogenic diet. This seasonal cycling kept their metabolism adaptable, a trait we can replicate today through intentional shifts in macronutrient intake."

To emulate these ancient patterns, consider alternating high-carb and low-carb days in your diet. On highcarb days, focus on fruits, root vegetables, and whole grains; on low-carb days, prioritize healthy fats and protein from sources like avocados, eggs, and grass-fed meats. This variation can help you develop metabolic flexibility while keeping your meals interesting and aligned with seasonal eating.

Section 6: Strategic Fasting

Fasting is the practice of intentionally abstaining from food for a specific period. While it may seem like a modern health trend, fasting has been a natural part of human history, stemming from the feast-andfamine cycles of our ancestors. Today, fasting is recognized for its ability to improve metabolic health, enhance cellular repair, and even promote longevity. Nowadays, you can visit a spa and spend a significant amount of money to have someone prevent you from eating.

Fasting works by triggering processes in the body that promote healing and repair. For example, during a fast, your body shifts from using glucose for energy to burning stored fat, which can lead to weight loss and improved metabolic health. Fasting also stimulates autophagy, a 'cellular cleaning' process where

damaged cells are broken down and recycled, reducing inflammation and lowering the risk of chronic diseases.

Incorporating fasting into your routine can enhance metabolic health, support fat burning, and stimulate cellular repair through processes like autophagy. Intermittent fasting has gained popularity in recent years, with many people achieving significant weight loss. However, for others, the thought of even skipping one meal feels daunting- almost as if the world might stop turning.

There are several types of fasting you can try:

•

Intermittent Fasting (16:8): Fast for 16 hours and eat during an 8-hour window.

•

Alternate-Day Fasting: Eat normally one day and restrict calories or fast completely the next.

•

Extended Fasting: Fast for 24-48 hours, typically done once a week or less.

Start with a method that feels manageable for you and adjust as you become more comfortable with fasting.

It's normal to feel a little hungry when you first try fasting, but most people find their bodies adapt quickly.

Staying hydrated and drinking herbal tea or black coffee can help curb hunger during a fast. If you feel lightheaded or unwell, it's okay to stop and try again later—fasting is a tool, not a requirement.

Fasting is a powerful way to reset your body and reconnect with its natural rhythms. Whether you start with a 12-hour fast or dive into intermittent fasting, you'll soon notice the benefits—clearer energy, better digestion, and even weight loss. Remember, fasting isn't about deprivation—it's about giving your body the space it needs to heal and thrive.

Chapter 7 – Living the Savage Life - Use of Oils, Wheat and Dairy (and why we do not use them) Part 1 Omega 6 vs Omega 3 Ratio

When humans were in a state of optimal health, the dietary ratio of Omega-6 to Omega-3 was approximately 1:1 to 4:1. This balance allowed for the proper functioning of inflammatory and antiinflammatory processes in the body. The Prehistoric diet was balanced at approximately 1:1 with Omega 6 vs Omega 3; which reflected a diet that was rich in wild game, fish, and foraged plants. This was when our immune system was intact and was considered very strong. The agricultural era shifted to around 4:1, including grains and reduced diversity in dietary fats. The Industrial Revolution raised the ratio to 10:1 with the introduction of refined oils and processed foods. Today, our modern diet has skyrocketed to 20:1 or higher, driven by seed oil consumption and a decline in omega-3 intake.

The dominance of Omega-6 fatty acids in modern diets promotes chronic inflammation, which is a root cause of many diseases, including heart disease, arthritis, and autoimmune disorders. Rebalancing this ratio by reducing processed oils and increasing Omega-3-rich foods like fatty fish and flaxseed can have a profound impact on health.

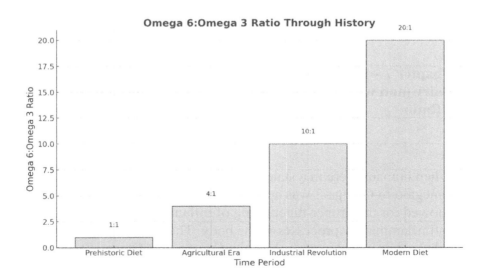

To restore balance, start by eliminating or reducing industrial seed oils from your diet. These include soybean oil, corn oil, sunflower oil, and cottonseed oil, which are commonly found in processed and packaged foods. Instead, cook with healthier fats like olive oil, coconut oil, or grass-fed butter. Incorporate Omega-3-rich foods like wild-caught salmon, sardines, and mackerel at least twice a week, and consider adding flaxseeds or walnuts to your meals.

I order specific laboratory tests from Vibrant Labs that provide clues about my patients' inflammation levels. I frequently order tests to assess markers of inflammation, such as C-reactive protein (CRP), Omega-6 to Omega-3 ratios in the blood, homocysteine, ferritin, sedimentation rate, and ESR. These tests offer valuable insights into how dietary imbalances impact overall health. If you're interested, ask your healthcare provider about testing your Omega-6 to Omega-3 ratio to gain a better understanding of your inflammatory state. The hunter-gatherer lifestyle was rich in Omega-3 from wild fish, game, plants, and grass-fed animals, while our current diet is far from healthy.

What is Omega 6?

So, what is Omega-6? Simply put, Omega-6 fatty acids, primarily derived from linoleic acid, are precursors to pro-inflammatory compounds. The Omega-3 fatty acids, like EPA and DHA, produce antiinflammatory and inflammation-resolving compounds. Both types of fats are essential, but the balance determines whether the body's inflammatory responses are regulated or excessive. In modern diets, Omega-6 dominance stems from industrial seed oils (e.g., soybean, corn, sunflower) and processed foods, combined with a decline in Omega-3 intake from sources like fatty fish and grass-fed meats.

Omega-6 is a family of polyunsaturated fatty acids (PUFAs) essential for human health. The body cannot produce Omega-6 fats, so they must be obtained through diet. Omega-6 fats play key roles in cellular function, inflammation, and energy production, but their effects depend on the balance with Omega-3 fats.

When Omega-6 fatty acids dominate the diet, they promote the production of inflammatory compounds called prostaglandins and cytokines. Over time, this chronic low-grade inflammation damages tissues and organs, contributing to conditions like heart disease, arthritis, and autoimmune disorders. In contrast,

Omega-3 fatty acids produce compounds that help resolve inflammation, keeping the body's immune response balanced and protecting against disease

What is Omega 3?

This is another family of essential polyunsaturated fats that support anti-inflammatory processes, brain health and cardiovascular function. The Alpha-linolenic (ALA) is found in flax seeds, chia seeds and walnuts. The other part of Omega 3 is Eicosapentaenoic acid (EPA)and Docosahexaenoic acid (DHA) which is found in fatty fish, fish oil, and algae. EPA has anti-inflammatory properties, and we have found that DHA is critical for both brain and eye health.

Comparison: Omega-6 vs. Omega-3

Aspect	Omega-6	Omega-3
Role in Body	Pro-inflammatory (in excess); aids healing, growth, and immune response.	Anti-inflammatory; supports brain health, cardiovascular health, and reduces chronic inflammation.
Sources	Vegetable oils (soybean, corn, sunflower), nuts, seeds, processed foods.	Fatty fish (salmon, mackerel, sardines), flaxseeds, walnuts, algae.
Balance in Diet	Excessive intake can lead to chronic inflammation.	Balances omega-6 effects, reducing inflammation

and supporting overall health.

Historical Ratio ~1:1 to 4:1 in ancestral diets. Balanced with omega-6 historically.

Modern

Often >10:1 to 20:1 due to processed

Ratio

food consumption.

Significantly out of balance in modern diets.

While achieving a perfect 1:1 ratio may be unrealistic in today's world, striving for a ratio of 4:1 or lower can significantly reduce inflammation and improve health. To do this, focus on reducing Omega-6 intake from processed foods and increasing Omega-3-rich foods in your diet.

The dominance of Omega-6 fatty acids in today's diet isn't just a historical accident—it's a health crisis.

By rebalancing your Omega-6 to Omega-3 ratio, you can take control of your health, reduce chronic inflammation, and align your diet with the principles of The Savage Diet. Begin today by eliminating processed seed oils, choosing healthier fats, and embracing foods rich in Omega-3s. Your body—and your future self—will thank you.

While the imbalance of Omega-6 to Omega-3 fatty acids is a major driver of inflammation, it's not the only modern dietary issue contributing to chronic disease. Next, we'll explore two other common staples of the modern diet—wheat and dairy—and why they no longer serve us as they once did."

Part 2 – The Wheat as we knew it

Over the centuries, wheat has transformed from a nutrient-dense staple of ancient diets into a highly processed, hybrid crop that promotes inflammation, spikes blood sugar, and contributes to nutrient

deficiencies. To understand why modern wheat no longer benefits us, we must examine how it has been fundamentally altered by hybridization, industrial farming, and the prioritization of yield over nutrition.

As the agricultural era has developed, the intake of Omega-6 fatty acids has increased due to higher consumption of grains and seeds, which has further increased the problem by the number of changes within the grains we have today. It has been hybridized and genetically modified to such a degree that one would have to question their sanity as to why they would eat it now.

For example, over the past 100 years, wheat has undergone extensive hybridization to improve yield, disease and pest resistance, and adaptability to various growing conditions. While these changes were designed to benefit agriculture, they have also significantly altered the nutritional profile and structure of wheat, which may have contributed to increased health issues like gluten sensitivity, inflammation, and metabolic disorders.

Wheat species like Einkorn, Emmer, and Spelt were grown for thousands of years. These had simpler genetic structures and lower gluten content. Einkorn has (14 chromosomes) and Emmer has (28

chromosomes) which were more nutrient-dense but less productive for our busy lifestyles. Today's dominant wheat is Triticum aestivum, a hexaploid species with 42 chromosomes, created through hybridization for greater productivity. Hybridization intensified after the mid-20th century with the development of dwarf wheat varieties. Wheat used to be very high, I remember walking through wheat fields as a child, it was nearly six feet tall. Today, we have shorter stalks so that the wheat will not fall over (lodging), or get eaten by rats and mice, putting it about 18 inches high. The Dwarf variety is sturdier, allowing more energy to be directed to grain production, and the short-stalked varieties could support heavier grain heads, which significantly increase the yield per acre. And then, for those of you who look at the end result, the Dwarf wheat varieties were bred to thrive with synthetic fertilizers. So, put that cherry on top. Today, over 99% of wheat grown globally is derived from these high-yield varieties.

Modern wheat has been hybridized repeatedly, with new genes and also increasing the genetic complexity, so the gluten protein in modern wheat has higher levels of gliadin, which makes it more inflammatory. It also has higher levels of amylopectin A, which is a type of starch associated with rapid blood sugar spikes. On the whole, I suppose the scientific community was looking to make our lives better, but hybridization has increased the traits for resistance to disease like rust, blight, and mildew, and it also caused complex genetic manipulations that altered the natural selections of wheat proteins. Which inadvertently causes changes within the wheat to make it harder for humans to digest. Prioritizing yield and disease resistance has come at a cost: the nutrient content of wheat has significantly declined. So, there are reductions in minerals like zinc, magnesium, and iron, and there is also a decline in fiber and protein quality. The effect is that modern wheat, which is all we have a choice of today is less nutrientdense than its ancient counterparts, which is leading to concerns about "hidden hunger" and micronutrient deficiencies. If you have a nutrient-poor diet, you will have a diet that is high in calories, usually mostly processed foods, with refined carbohydrates. What I find with my patients is that those who only cook at home usually will eat the same type of foods week after week. Those who eat out will do the same type of restaurant-cooked meals or fast food meals, which puts them at a higher risk for increased inflammation. However, patients who stay at home and eat the same type of meals are at an increased risk of very low gut diversity. Both are at risk for different health concerns.

The wheat we consume today is a far cry from the nutrient-dense grains our ancestors relied on for sustenance. By prioritizing yield and disease resistance over nutrition, we've created a food that contributes to chronic inflammation, metabolic dysfunction, and nutrient deficiencies. To live in alignment with the principles of The Savage Diet, we must reconsider our reliance on modern wheat and embrace more diverse, nutrient-dense alternatives.

A 2008 study published in the Journal of Agricultural and Food Chemistry found that modern wheat varieties contain 30-40% less zinc and iron compared to varieties grown in the mid-20th century. Similarly,

the prevalence of celiac disease has quadrupled over the past 50 years, paralleling the rise in hybridized wheat consumption.

To reduce the impact of modern wheat on your health, try incorporating ancient grains like Einkorn, Spelt, or Emmer into your meals. These grains are less inflammatory and more nutrient-dense than modern wheat. If you're sensitive to gluten or looking to reduce blood sugar spikes, consider replacing wheat with gluten-free options like quinoa, buckwheat, or root vegetables such as sweet potatoes. Additionally, aim to diversify your diet by rotating different foods each week to promote a healthy gut microbiome.

Part 3: The perfect storm....How this affects our health

The increased gluten content and altered protein structure may have (likely) contributed to the rise in gluten intolerance and celiac disease. When you have gliadin, which is a component of gluten, this can trigger a strong immune response in sensitive individuals (everybody). I postulate, that over time, the response may not be felt as per se, but is still influencing how much microbiome dysbiosis and/or inflammation is occurring. In my clinic, I've observed that many patients don't notice symptoms like gas or bloating until they remove wheat from their diet. They then re-introduce the culprit food, and they feel significant pain, bloating, and sometimes nausea. High amylopectin A in modern wheat leads to rapid blood sugar spikes, which has contributed to obesity, type 2 diabetes, and metabolic syndrome.

Hybridization has increased inflammation, contributing to a global rise in autoimmune conditions.

The higher gliadin content in modern wheat increases gluten's inflammatory potential, which can contribute to gut permeability ('leaky gut') and trigger immune responses in susceptible individuals. This may explain the rise in gluten sensitivity and autoimmune conditions like celiac disease. Leaky gut occurs when the lining of the intestinal wall becomes more permeable than it should be, allowing undigested food particles, toxins, and microbes to pass into the bloodstream. Gliadin, a component of gluten, has been shown to increase gut permeability in sensitive individuals by triggering the release of zonulin, a protein that loosens tight junctions in the gut lining. Over time, this can lead to chronic inflammation, food sensitivities, and autoimmune reactions."

Comparison of Wheat Varieties

Aspect	Ancient Wheat (Einkorn, Emmer)	Modern Wheat (Dwarf Varieties)
Height	Tall (4–5 feet)	Short (2–3 feet)
Chromosomes	Simple (14–28 chromosomes)	Complex (42 chromosomes)
Yield	Low	High
Gluten Content	Lower, simpler gluten structure	Higher, more complex gluten structure
Nutrient Density	High	Reduced

Disease Resistance Low

High

So, why? The hybridization of wheat over the past century has fundamentally changed its genetic makeup, its nutritional profile, and its effects on human health. While these changes improved agricultural productivity and global food security, they also introduced far greater challenges, including reduced nutrient density and potential health risks. Understanding these changes is key to making informed dietary choices and exploring alternatives like ancient grains or heirloom wheat varieties. It is also about saying no. Try your own products at home that are more in keeping with being like the caveman of today.

Look through the recipes that I have made into the book to make your own recipes or order the workbook at www.thesavage diet.com. I would also ask myself if mice and rats won't eat this product, should I?

The Ancient wheat had simpler genomes 14-28, while our modern wheat has a complex genome of 42

chromosomes. Ancient wheat also had a simpler and lower gluten content, making it easier to digest, and the nutrient density was much richer in nutrients compared to modern wheat. The only thing our modern wheat is bred for is its higher productivity and its resistance to pests. Now, is this really Ancient? We only began to cultivate wheat on any type of scale about 9000 BCE or 10,000 years ago. This period marked our transition from nomadic hunter-gatherer societies to settled agricultural communities.

Modern wheat is not the wheat our ancestors ate. Its increased gluten content, altered protein structure, and high levels of amylopectin A have created a perfect storm of health challenges. From rising rates of gluten intolerance and celiac disease to obesity, type 2 diabetes, and autoimmune conditions, the effects of hybridized wheat on human health are profound. Understanding these changes is the first step toward reclaiming our health.

Part 4: Globalization

The expansion of fast food chains globally that is standardized by a diet high in calories, fats, and sugars, further distancing eating habits from traditional, whole-food based diets has changed the world and our global health. The rise of convenience foods also introduced a flood of processed ingredients into the average diet—refined sugars, artificial flavors, preservatives, and industrial seed oils. These ingredients were designed for shelf stability, not nutrition, fundamentally altering the way people thought about and consumed food. Over time, home cooking and traditional recipes were replaced by pre-packaged meals and drive-thru options, creating a profound disconnect between people and their food.

Convenience foods not only changed what we eat but also how we eat. Family meals gave way to graband-go snacks, and the once-standard practice of cooking at home became a weekend hobby rather than a daily necessity. This shift has eroded the cultural and emotional significance of shared meals, replacing them with hurried bites consumed in front of a screen or on the way to the next obligation.

In the 1950s, TV dinners became a household staple, with Salisbury steak and mashed potatoes served in foil trays that could be heated in the oven. By the 1970s, boxed macaroni and cheese and instant ramen provided cheap, quick options for busy families. By the 1990s, grocery store aisles were filled with frozen entrees promising restaurant-quality meals in under 5 minutes, further distancing consumers from fresh, whole foods. I thought back to when I was young and what my Mother fed us kids and how we ate.

I do remember TV dinners for a short period of time, and I remember it was Salisbury steak, of all things.

Then, I believe my Mother tired of that type of food because, after that short period of time, we never had TV dinners again. There was never a McDonald's in my life until I graduated high school and was out on my own. I feel I was lucky at that point, because the U.S. Navy sent me to isolated islands around the world, or to countries that did not have McDonalds or anything resembling fast food.

Advertising campaigns painted convenience foods as symbols of progress and modernity, appealing to busy families with promises of ease and efficiency. Slogans like McDonald's 'You deserve a break today'

reinforced the idea that cooking from scratch was an unnecessary burden. Meanwhile, low-fat and dietfocused products were marketed as healthy alternatives, creating confusion about what truly constituted a nourishing meal.

So, the transition to a modern diet was driven by a complex interplay of technological advancements, agricultural developments, economic changes, and social transformations. This diet, while increasing food availability and convenience, has also been linked to the rise of non-communicable diseases such as obesity, diabetes, heart disease, and other health issues. We are becoming more aware of these impacts, and I believe that there is a growing movement to return to diets that emphasize whole, minimally processed foods, much like the principles in "The Savage Diet".

Part 5: Convenience

As we discussed in earlier chapters, during World War II, there was a significant increase in the production of pre-packaged and convenience foods. Innovations such as frozen foods, instant coffee, and microwave meals emerged, catering to the growing number of dual-income households and the desire for quick and easy meal solutions. The mid-20th century saw the rise of fast food culture, with chains like McDonald's pioneering a model built on speed, consistency, and low cost. This revolutionized how Americans ate, prioritizing convenience over nutrition. By the 1970s and 1980s, there was growing public awareness about the health impacts of diet, and this led to the introduction of diet-specific and healthoriented products, including low-fat, low-sugar, and later, low-carb options and everything else you could imagine to be used as "food". I often ask my patients if they're on the 'low fat, no fat, don't even think about fat' diet—a belief that, unfortunately, remains deeply ingrained despite its flaws.

Unfortunately, I hear way too often how they are avoiding fats because out of all of the things the internet has brought to them, that is what they have clung to, to avoid fat.

The low-fat diet craze of the 1980s and 1990s was fueled by flawed science and aggressive marketing, convincing millions that dietary fat was the enemy of health. This led to an explosion of 'fat-free' and

'lowfat' products loaded with sugar and refined carbohydrates to compensate for the loss of flavor. The result was a generation of people avoiding healthy fats—like those in avocados, nuts, and olive oil—that are essential for hormone production, brain health, and satiety.

The rise of convenience foods promised a simpler, more efficient way of life, but it came at a cost: the erosion of our connection to real, nourishing food. To reclaim our health, we must push back against the convenience culture, prioritize whole ingredients, and rediscover the joy of preparing and sharing meals.

Convenience doesn't have to mean sacrificing nutrition—it can mean finding simple ways to honor our bodies and the ancestral wisdom that guided our diets for millennia.

In today's busy world, avoiding convenience foods altogether may seem unrealistic. Instead, focus on small, manageable changes. Try meal prepping on Sundays to have healthy options ready for the week, or start replacing one processed snack with a piece of fruit or a handful of nuts. Cooking simple, wholefood meals doesn't have to be complicated—a roasted chicken and a tray of vegetables can provide multiple meals with minimal effort.

Chapter 8: The Savage Recipes

Here is the heart of The Savage Diet – where nourishment meets simplicity. In this section, you will find a collection of recipes designed to fuel your body with nutrient-dense, whole foods that align with our ancestral way of eating. We embrace the wisdom of nature by focusing on unprocessed, wholesome ingredients while eliminating the common culprits that have infiltrated modern diets.

Each recipe is crafted to support your health, enhance digestion, and nourish your body in a way that's both satisfying and sustainable. By stepping away from the conventional use of grains, oils, and dairy, we focus on nutrient-rich vegetables, healthy fats from animal sources, lean proteins and natural foods that have sustained us for millennia.

Section 1: Cooking Tips

1. • Prepare and cook in batches to save time. For example, batch-cook proteins like chicken, beef, or pork and store them in the fridge or freezer for quick meal assembly throughout the week.

•

Storage Tips: Keep cooked meats, vegetables, and salads in glass airtight containers to maintain freshness for several days.

2. Cooking Methods and Substitutions •

Healthy Fats for Cooking: It is important that you are

choosing healthy fats to cook with. These fats support nutrient absorption and enhance the flavor of meals.

•

Grain-Free Alternatives: How to substitute common grains (like rice or pasta) with alternatives such as cauliflower rice, zucchini noodles, or spaghetti squash. This helps make meals more in line with The Savage Diet. Always look for any kind of pastas made directly in Italy. This is very important, they do not treat their wheat the same as we do here in the United States, and people have much fewer gut issues when they eat their pasta.

3. Fermented Foods Usage

•

Add fermented foods (such as kimchi, sauerkraut, and kefir) to each meal to support gut health.

4. Food Preparation for Families

•

Adapting Recipes for Families: Adapting recipes to suit larger families, like making double batches, or using one main protein (e.g., a roast) that can be served in multiple ways throughout the week.

•

Kid-Friendly Modifications: Modifying meals to make them more palatable for kids while still staying true to the diet principles. For example, turning a salad into a wrap or using "hidden"

vegetables in a meatball mixture.

5. Making Meals Travel-Friendly

-

Portable Meal Ideas: These meals can be packed for work, school, or travel. For example, you can prepare mason jar salads, pre-made smoothie packs, or protein-packed snack bars.

-

Lunchbox Tips: Here are easy-to-carry meals that are portable and nutritious, such as hard-boiled eggs, vegetable sticks with dip, or roasted meats with a side of raw vegetables.

6. Adjusting Recipes for Special Needs

-

Customizing for Dietary Restrictions: These recipes are suitable for other dietary restrictions (such as dairy-free, nut-free, etc.) while staying within the confines of The Savage Diet. For example, coconut yogurt or avocado instead of dairy-based options.

7. Seasonings and Flavor Enhancements

-

Herbs and Spices: Experiment with a variety of fresh herbs, spices, and flavorings to make meals more exciting and diverse. Offer suggestions for commonly used herbs and spices, such as turmeric, cumin, rosemary, thyme, or ginger, and their health benefits.

- Homemade Dressings and Sauces: You will find simple homemade dressings and sauces (e.g., tahini dressing, avocado-based mayo, or coconut aminos) to complement meals without relying on store-bought options that may contain unhealthy additives or sugars.

8. Portion Control and Meal Planning

- Meal Portioning: Always think of mindful portioning, focusing on balanced meals with adequate protein, healthy fats, and vegetables.

- Meal Timing: If you are following the Savage Diet then this is a way of intermittent fasting.

9. Seasonal and Local Ingredients

- Cooking with Seasons: Use seasonally and locally-sourced produce in recipes to keep meals fresh and varied throughout the year. A seasonal ingredients list can also encourage sustainability and cost-effectiveness.

- Farmer's Market Tips: Shop at the local farmer's markets or directly from farmers to get the best, freshest options for vegetables, meats, and dairy.

10. Hydration and Detox Tips

-

Drinks and Hydration: At the end of this Chapter, you will find easy-to-prepare, diet-compliant drinks such as herbal teas, water with lemon, or bone broth. You must stay hydrated the importance of staying hydrated while following the diet.

-

Detox Support: Provide tips for incorporating detox-friendly foods (like leafy greens, cruciferous vegetables, and lemon water) into meals to support the body's natural detox processes.

Section 2: Savage Recipes

Day 1

Breakfast: Savory Egg and Avocado Bowl

Ingredients:

-

2 eggs (fried or scrambled in grass-fed butter)

-

1/2 avocado, sliced

-

1/2 cup sautéed spinach or kale

•

1/4 cup fermented vegetables (such as sauerkraut or kimchi)

•

Salt and pepper, to taste

•

Optional: Sprinkle of chia seeds or flaxseeds for added fiber
Instructions:

1. In a skillet, sauté the spinach or kale in some butter until wilted.

2. While that's cooking, fry or scramble the eggs in butter.

3. Assemble your bowl by adding the sautéed spinach, eggs, avocado slices, and fermented vegetables.

4. Top with chia seeds or flaxseeds if desired and season with salt and pepper.

Benefits: This meal is rich in healthy fats, protein, and fiber, promoting satiety and good digestion. The fermented vegetables also support gut health.

Lunch: Grilled Chicken Salad with Nutty Dressing

• •

-
-

Ingredients:

1 chicken breast (grilled or roasted)

2 cups mixed greens (spinach, arugula, or lettuce)

1/4 cup sliced almonds or walnuts

1/4 cup cucumber, sliced

-

1/4 cup cherry tomatoes, halved

-

1 tablespoon olive oil

-

1 tablespoon apple cider vinegar

-

1 teaspoon Dijon mustard

-

Salt and pepper to taste

Instructions:

1. Grill or roast the chicken breast and slice it into strips.

2. Toss the mixed greens, cucumber, cherry tomatoes, and nuts in a bowl.

3. In a small bowl, whisk together olive oil, apple cider vinegar, mustard, salt, and pepper for the dressing.

4. Drizzle the dressing over the salad and top with the sliced chicken.

Benefits: A nutrient-dense salad rich in protein, fiber, and heart-healthy fats. The addition of nuts offers a crunch while providing omega-3s and other healthy fats.

Dinner: Beef Stir-Fry with Veggies

Ingredients:

•

1/2 lb grass-fed beef, thinly sliced

•

1 cup broccoli florets

•

1 bell pepper, sliced

•

1 small zucchini, sliced

•

1 tablespoon coconut oil or olive oil

•

1 tablespoon coconut aminos (a soy sauce alternative)

•

1 tablespoon minced garlic

•

1 teaspoon ginger, grated

•

1 tablespoon sesame seeds

•

Optional: 1/4 avocado, sliced

Instructions:

1. Heat oil in a large skillet or wok over medium-high heat.

2. Add garlic and ginger, and sauté for 1 minute until fragrant.

3. Add the sliced beef and stir-fry until browned.

4. Toss in the broccoli, bell pepper, and zucchini, cooking until tender.

5. Stir in the coconut aminos and cook for an additional minute. 6. Serve the stir-fry topped with sesame seeds and optional avocado slices.

Benefits: Packed with protein and fiber, this dish is also high in vitamins and antioxidants from the colorful veggies. Coconut aminos add flavor without grains or soy.

Day 2

Breakfast: Bacon and Spinach Frittata

Ingredients:

- 4 eggs

- 2 slices bacon, chopped

- 1 cup spinach, chopped

- 1/4 onion, diced

- 1 tablespoon ghee or butter

- Salt and pepper to taste

Instructions:

1. Heat ghee or butter in an oven-safe pan and cook bacon until crispy.

2. Add onions and spinach, cooking until softened.

3. In a bowl, whisk eggs, then pour over the cooked bacon and spinach. 4. Transfer the pan to the oven and bake at 375°F for 15–20 minutes until eggs are set.

Benefits: A protein-packed breakfast full of healthy fats, greens, and flavor.

Lunch: Beef and Avocado Lettuce Wraps

Ingredients:

•

1/2 lb ground beef

•

1/4 onion, diced

•

1 avocado, sliced

•

4-6 large lettuce leaves (for wraps)

•

1 tablespoon olive oil

•

Salt, pepper, and chili powder to taste

Instructions:

1. In a skillet, cook ground beef with onions until browned.

2. Season with salt, pepper, and chili powder.

3. Assemble the wraps by placing the beef mixture and avocado slices into the lettuce leaves.

4. Serve with a side of fermented veggies like kimchi or sauerkraut.

Benefits: A low-carb, high-protein lunch with healthy fats and fiber from the avocado and lettuce.

Dinner: Grilled Shrimp with Zucchini Noodles

Ingredients:

•

1/2 lb shrimp, peeled and deveined

-

2 zucchinis, spiralized into noodles

-

1 tablespoon olive oil

-

1 tablespoon garlic, minced

-

1/4 cup fresh parsley, chopped

-

Salt, pepper, and lemon juice to taste

Instructions:

1. Grill shrimp until pink and cooked through.

2. In a skillet, sauté zucchini noodles in olive oil and garlic for 3-4 minutes until tender.

3. Toss shrimp with the zucchini noodles and garnish with fresh parsley, salt, pepper, and lemon juice.

- •

-

-

Benefits: A light yet filling dinner full of protein and low-carb vegetables, perfect for digestion.

Day 3

Breakfast: Smoked Salmon and Avocado Salad Ingredients:

•

2 oz smoked salmon

•

1/2 avocado, sliced

2 cups mixed greens (arugula, spinach)

1 tablespoon olive oil

1 tablespoon lemon juice Salt

and pepper to taste

Instructions:

1. Toss mixed greens with olive oil, lemon juice, salt, and pepper.

2. Top with smoked salmon and avocado slices.

Benefits: A high-protein, omega-3-rich breakfast that supports heart health and energy levels.

Lunch: Turkey and Veggie Lettuce Wraps

Ingredients:

-

4 oz turkey breast, sliced

-

4-6 large lettuce leaves (for wraps)

-

1/4 cucumber, thinly sliced

-

1/4 avocado, sliced

-

1 tablespoon mustard or olive oil mayo

Instructions:

1. Lay lettuce leaves flat and layer with turkey, cucumber, avocado, and mustard or mayo.

2. Roll up the lettuce wraps and enjoy.

Benefits: A light yet filling lunch with lean protein, healthy fats, and fiber from veggies.

Dinner: Grilled Steak with Roasted Asparagus

Ingredients:

-

1 steak (ribeye, sirloin, or your choice)

-

1 bunch asparagus

-

2 tablespoons olive oil

-

Salt, pepper, and garlic powder to taste

Instructions:

1. Preheat the grill and cook the steak to your desired doneness.

2. Toss asparagus in olive oil, salt, pepper, and garlic powder. Roast at 400°F for 10-15 minutes until tender.

3. Serve the steak with roasted asparagus on the side.

Benefits: A protein-heavy dinner with nutrient-dense vegetables, providing fullness and strength.

Day 4

Breakfast: Chia Seed Pudding with Nuts and Berries

Ingredients:

-

1/4 cup chia seeds

-

1 cup unsweetened coconut milk (or almond milk)

-

1 teaspoon vanilla extract

-

1 tablespoon almond butter

-

1/4 cup mixed berries (blueberries, raspberries, or strawberries)

-

1 tablespoon mixed nuts (almonds, walnuts, pecans)

Instructions:

1. In a bowl, mix chia seeds, coconut milk, and vanilla extract. Stir well and refrigerate overnight.

2. In the morning, top with almond butter, mixed berries, and nuts.

Benefits: A high-fiber, omega-3-rich breakfast that promotes digestive health and keeps you full throughout the morning.

Lunch: Chicken and Avocado Salad with Olive Oil Dressing

Ingredients:

·

1 grilled chicken breast, sliced

·

2 cups mixed greens (spinach, arugula, etc.)

·

1/2 avocado, sliced

·

1/4 cucumber, sliced

·

1 tablespoon olive oil

·

1 tablespoon apple cider vinegar

-

Salt and pepper to taste

Instructions:

1. Toss the mixed greens, cucumber, and avocado in a bowl.

2. Drizzle with olive oil, apple cider vinegar, salt, and pepper.

3. Top with sliced grilled chicken.

Benefits: A protein-packed salad with healthy fats from avocado and olive oil, perfect for balancing blood sugar and supporting healthy digestion.

Dinner: Baked Lemon Herb Chicken with Roasted Cauliflower

Ingredients:

-

2 chicken thighs, bone-in, skin-on

-

1 tablespoon olive oil

-

1 teaspoon dried oregano

-

1 teaspoon garlic powder

-

1/2 teaspoon paprika

-

1 lemon (zested and juiced)

-

2 cups cauliflower florets

-

Salt and pepper to taste

- -
-
-

Instructions:

1. Preheat the oven to 400°F (200°C).

2. Rub the chicken thighs with olive oil, oregano, garlic powder, paprika, lemon zest, and salt and pepper. Bake for 30–35 minutes until the skin is crispy and the chicken is cooked through.

3. Toss cauliflower florets with olive oil, salt, and pepper, and roast for 20–25 minutes until tender.

4. Serve the chicken with roasted cauliflower.

Benefits: A satisfying dinner with protein, healthy fats, and cruciferous vegetables that support detoxification and gut health.

Day 5

Breakfast: Turkey Bacon and Veggie Omelette

Ingredients:

2 eggs

2 slices turkey bacon, chopped

1/2 cup mushrooms, sliced

1/4 onion, diced

•

1/4 cup spinach, chopped

•

1 tablespoon olive oil or butter

•

Salt and pepper to taste

Instructions:

1. Cook the turkey bacon in a pan until crispy. Remove and set aside.

2. In the same pan, sauté the mushrooms, onions, and spinach in olive oil or butter until softened.

3. Whisk eggs in a bowl and pour into the pan, cooking until set. Add turkey bacon and vegetables to one side and fold the omelette over.

4. Serve warm with a sprinkle of salt and pepper.

Benefits: A protein and veggie-packed breakfast to start your day with energy and fullness.

Lunch: Tuna Salad with Olive Oil and Pickles

Ingredients:

-

1 can of tuna in olive oil (drained)

-

1/4 cup diced pickles (dill or fermented)

-

1 tablespoon olive oil

-

1 tablespoon lemon juice

-

1 tablespoon Dijon mustard

-

Salt and pepper to taste

-

2 cups mixed greens (arugula, spinach, etc.)

Instructions:

1. In a bowl, combine tuna, pickles, olive oil, lemon juice, Dijon mustard, salt, and pepper. 2.

Serve the tuna salad over mixed greens for a light, satisfying meal.

Benefits: Rich in omega-3 fatty acids and protein, this meal promotes heart health and helps keep you full.

Dinner: Grilled Lamb Chops with Broccoli Slaw

Ingredients:

-

2 lamb chops

-

1 tablespoon olive oil

-

1 teaspoon rosemary, chopped

•

Salt and pepper to taste

•

2 cups broccoli slaw (pre-made or homemade with shredded broccoli, carrots, and cabbage)

•

1 tablespoon apple cider vinegar

•

1 tablespoon olive oil

•

Salt and pepper to taste

Instructions:

1. Preheat the grill and season lamb chops with olive oil, rosemary, salt, and pepper. Grill for about 4-5 minutes per side.

2. Toss broccoli slaw with apple cider vinegar, olive oil, salt, and pepper.

3. Serve the lamb chops with the slaw on the side.

Benefits: A delicious, hearty dinner with protein, fiber, and healthy fats that promote satiety and overall health.

Day 6

- •

- •

- •

Breakfast: Smoked Salmon and Avocado Scramble

Ingredients:

-

2 eggs

-

2 oz smoked salmon, chopped

-

1/2 avocado, diced

-

1 tablespoon ghee or butter

-

Salt and pepper to taste

-

Fresh dill (optional)

Instructions:

1. Heat ghee or butter in a pan, scramble the eggs until cooked through.

2. Add smoked salmon and diced avocado, stirring to combine.

3. Top with fresh dill, salt, and pepper.

Benefits: Omega-3-rich and high in protein, this breakfast promotes brain health and provides a satisfying start to the day.

Lunch: Shrimp and Avocado Salad

Ingredients:

•

6 oz shrimp, cooked and peeled

•

2 cups mixed greens (spinach, arugula)

•

1/2 avocado, diced

•

1/4 red onion, thinly sliced

•

1 tablespoon olive oil

•

1 tablespoon lime juice

•

Salt and pepper to taste

Instructions:

1. Toss mixed greens, avocado, red onion, and shrimp in a bowl.

2. Drizzle with olive oil, lime juice, salt, and pepper.

Benefits: A light, refreshing lunch packed with protein, healthy fats, and fiber.

Dinner: Grilled Steak with Sweet Potato and Greens

Ingredients:

•

1 ribeye steak (or preferred cut)

•

1 medium sweet potato, roasted

•

1 cup sautéed spinach or kale

-

1 tablespoon olive oil

-

Salt and pepper to taste

Instructions:

1. Grill steak to your preferred level of doneness.

2. Roast sweet potato at 400°F (200°C) for 30-40 minutes until soft.

3. Sauté spinach or kale in olive oil until wilted and season with salt and pepper.

4. Serve steak with roasted sweet potato and sautéed greens.

Benefits: A protein and fiber-rich dinner that provides energy and supports muscle recovery.

Day 7:

Breakfast: Sweet Potato and Bacon Hash with Eggs

Ingredients:

-

1 medium sweet potato, peeled and diced

-

2 slices of bacon, chopped

-

1/4 onion, diced

-

1/2 bell pepper, diced

-

2 eggs

-

1 tablespoon olive oil or ghee

-

Salt and pepper to taste

-

Fresh parsley for garnish (optional)

Instructions:

1. Heat the olive oil or ghee in a skillet over medium heat.

2. Add the chopped bacon and cook until crispy, then remove from the pan and set aside.

3. In the same pan, add the diced sweet potato and cook for 8-10 minutes until tender and slightly caramelized.

4. Add the onion and bell pepper, sautéing until softened.

5. Push the mixture to the side and crack two eggs into the pan, cooking them to your desired level of doneness.

6. Top the sweet potato hash with crispy bacon and serve with the eggs. Garnish with fresh parsley.

Benefits: Sweet potatoes provide complex carbs and fiber, bacon adds healthy fats and flavor, and eggs offer protein to kickstart your day.

Lunch: Zucchini and Ground Beef Stir-Fry with Coconut Aminos
Ingredients:

•

1/2 lb grass-fed ground beef

•

2 medium zucchinis, sliced into half-moons

•

1 tablespoon coconut oil

•

2 tablespoons coconut aminos (or tamari for a soy-free option)

-

1 garlic clove, minced

-

1/2 teaspoon ginger, grated

-

1 tablespoon sesame seeds (optional)

-

Salt and pepper to taste

Instructions:

1. Heat the coconut oil in a skillet over medium heat.

2. Add the ground beef and cook until browned, breaking it apart as it cooks.

3. Add the garlic and ginger, cooking for 1-2 minutes until fragrant.

4. Toss in the zucchini and cook for 4-5 minutes until tender but still slightly crisp.

5. Drizzle with coconut aminos, and stir well to coat. Season with salt and pepper to taste.

6. Sprinkle sesame seeds on top and serve.

Benefits: This stir-fry is loaded with protein and fiber, with healthy fats from coconut oil and sesame seeds. The zucchini adds valuable nutrients without any grains.

Dinner: Lemon Herb Chicken Thighs with Cauliflower Rice

Ingredients:

-

2 bone-in, skin-on chicken thighs

-

1 tablespoon olive oil

-

1 teaspoon fresh thyme, chopped (or 1/2 teaspoon dried thyme)

-

1 tablespoon fresh lemon juice

-

1 garlic clove, minced

-

1/2 medium head of cauliflower, grated into rice-sized pieces (or use a food processor)

-

1 tablespoon ghee or coconut oil

•

Salt and pepper to taste

Instructions:

1. Preheat the oven to 400°F (200°C).

2. Rub the chicken thighs with olive oil, thyme, lemon juice, garlic, salt, and pepper.

3. Place the chicken on a baking sheet and roast for 30-35 minutes, or until the skin is crispy and the chicken is cooked through.

4. While the chicken is baking, prepare the cauliflower rice: Heat ghee or coconut oil in a large pan over medium heat.

5. Add the grated cauliflower and sauté for 5-7 minutes until tender and lightly golden.

6. Season the cauliflower rice with salt and pepper, and serve alongside the roasted chicken.

Benefits: This meal provides healthy fats from ghee, protein from chicken, and fiber from cauliflower, making it a satisfying and nutrient-dense dinner.

Day 8

Breakfast: Scrambled Eggs with Spinach and Avocado

Ingredients:

- 3 eggs

- 1/2 avocado, sliced

- 1 cup spinach

- 1 tablespoon olive oil or butter

- Salt and pepper to taste

Instructions:

1. Heat olive oil or butter in a pan and sauté spinach until wilted.

2. Crack the eggs into the pan, scrambling them with the spinach.

3. Season with salt and pepper, and top with sliced avocado.

Benefits: A balanced meal with protein, healthy fats, and vegetables to start the day.

Lunch: Grilled Chicken Salad with Avocado and Fermented Vegetables Ingredients:

- 1 grilled chicken breast, sliced

- 2 cups mixed greens (arugula, spinach, or lettuce)

- 1/2 avocado, sliced

- 1/4 cup fermented vegetables (kimchi or sauerkraut)

- 1 tablespoon olive oil

- 1 tablespoon apple cider vinegar

- Salt and pepper to taste

Instructions:

1. Toss mixed greens, avocado, and fermented vegetables in a bowl.

2. Top with grilled chicken and drizzle with olive oil and apple cider vinegar.

3. Season with salt and pepper.

Benefits: High in protein and healthy fats, this salad also provides gut-friendly probiotics from the fermented vegetables.

Dinner: Baked Salmon with Roasted Brussels Sprouts

Ingredients:

•

1 salmon fillet

•

2 cups Brussels sprouts, halved

•

1 tablespoon olive oil

•

1 teaspoon garlic powder

•

Salt and pepper to taste

Instructions:

1. Preheat the oven to 400°F (200°C).

2. Toss Brussels sprouts with olive oil, garlic powder, salt, and pepper. Roast for 25-30 minutes.

3. Season the salmon with salt and pepper and bake for 12-15 minutes until cooked through.

4. Serve the salmon with roasted Brussels sprouts.

Benefits: Omega-3-rich salmon paired with fiber-rich Brussels sprouts for a heart-healthy and satisfying dinner.

Day 9

Breakfast: Chia Seed Pudding with Berries

Ingredients:

-

1/4 cup chia seeds

-

1 cup unsweetened coconut milk (or almond milk)

-

1 teaspoon vanilla extract

-

1/4 cup mixed berries

-

1 tablespoon almonds or walnuts, chopped

Instructions:

1. Mix chia seeds, coconut milk, and vanilla extract in a jar or bowl. Refrigerate overnight.

2. In the morning, top with fresh berries and chopped nuts.

Benefits: Chia seeds provide fiber and omega-3s, while the berries offer antioxidants.

Lunch: Turkey Lettuce Wraps

Ingredients:

-

4-6 large lettuce leaves

-

6 oz sliced turkey breast

-

1/2 avocado, sliced

-

1/4 cup sliced cucumber

•

1 tablespoon mustard or olive oil mayo

Instructions:

1. Lay out the lettuce leaves and top with turkey, avocado, cucumber, and mustard or mayo.

2. Wrap the lettuce leaves around the filling and serve.

Benefits: Low in carbs and high in protein and healthy fats, this meal is easy to prepare and satisfying Dinner: Beef Stir-Fry with Vegetables

Ingredients:

•

1/2 lb grass-fed beef, thinly sliced

•

1 cup broccoli florets

•

1 bell pepper, sliced

•

1 small zucchini, sliced

-

2 tablespoons coconut oil or olive oil

-

1 tablespoon coconut aminos

-

1 teaspoon garlic, minced

-

Salt and pepper to taste

Instructions:

1. Heat coconut oil in a pan, and cook garlic until fragrant.

2. Add beef and cook until browned.

3. Toss in the broccoli, bell pepper, and zucchini, and stir-fry for 5-7 minutes.

4. Drizzle with coconut aminos and season with salt and pepper.

Benefits: A colorful, nutrient-packed stir-fry with protein and fiber-rich vegetables for a well-rounded meal.

Day 10

Breakfast: Bacon and Vegetable Frittata

Ingredients:

- 4 eggs

- 2 slices bacon, chopped

- 1/2 cup mushrooms, sliced

- 1/2 cup spinach, chopped

- 1 tablespoon ghee or butter

- Salt and pepper to taste

Instructions:

1. Heat ghee or butter in an oven-safe pan, and cook bacon until crispy.

2. Add mushrooms and spinach, cooking until softened.

3. Whisk the eggs, pour them over the veggies, and bake at 375°F (190°C) for 10-12 minutes until set.

4. Season with salt and pepper.

Benefits: A protein-packed breakfast with healthy fats and greens.

Lunch: Grilled Shrimp Salad with Lemon Vinaigrette

Ingredients:

-

1/2 lb shrimp, peeled and deveined

-

2 cups mixed greens (spinach, arugula, etc.)

-

1/4 cup cucumber, sliced

-

1/4 red onion, thinly sliced

-

1 tablespoon olive oil

-

1 tablespoon lemon juice

-

Salt and pepper to taste

Instructions:

1. Grill the shrimp until pink and cooked through.

2. Toss mixed greens, cucumber, and red onion with olive oil and lemon juice.

3. Top with shrimp and season with salt and pepper.

Benefits: This light and refreshing salad is high in protein, antioxidants, and healthy fats.

Dinner: Roast Chicken with Sweet Potatoes

Ingredients:

-

2 chicken thighs, bone-in, skin-on

-

1 medium sweet potato, diced

-

2 tablespoons olive oil

-

1 tablespoon rosemary, chopped

-

Salt and pepper to taste

Instructions:

1. Preheat the oven to 400°F (200°C).

2. Toss sweet potato with olive oil, rosemary, salt, and pepper, and roast for 20-25 minutes.

3. Season chicken thighs with salt and pepper, and roast for 35-40 minutes until golden and cooked through.

4. Serve chicken with roasted sweet potatoes.

Benefits: High in protein and healthy carbs, this meal provides steady energy throughout the evening.

Day 11

Breakfast: Smoothie with Coconut Milk and Berries

Ingredients:

•

1/2 cup unsweetened coconut milk

•

1/2 cup mixed berries

-

1/2 avocado

-

1 tablespoon chia seeds

-

1 scoop protein powder (optional)

Instructions:

1. Blend all ingredients in a blender until smooth.

2. Pour into a glass and serve.

Benefits: This smoothie is packed with healthy fats, antioxidants, and fiber, making it a great way to fuel your day.

Lunch: Salmon Salad with Cucumber and Dill

Ingredients:

-

1 salmon fillet, grilled or baked

-

2 cups mixed greens

•

1/2 cucumber, sliced

•

1 tablespoon fresh dill, chopped

•

1 tablespoon olive oil

•

1 tablespoon lemon juice

•

Salt and pepper to taste

Instructions:

1. Grill or bake the salmon until cooked through.

2. Toss mixed greens, cucumber, and dill in a bowl.

3. Drizzle with olive oil and lemon juice, and top with salmon.

Benefits: Rich in omega-3 fatty acids, this meal supports heart and brain health.

Dinner: Pork Tenderloin with Roasted Vegetables

Ingredients:

-

1 pork tenderloin

-

1 cup carrots, sliced

-

1 cup Brussels sprouts, halved

-

2 tablespoons olive oil

-

Salt and pepper to taste

Instructions:

1. Preheat the oven to 400°F (200°C).

2. Rub pork tenderloin with olive oil, salt, and pepper. Roast for 25-30 minutes until cooked through.

3. Toss carrots and Brussels sprouts with olive oil, salt, and pepper. Roast for 20-25 minutes.

4. Serve the pork with roasted vegetables.

Benefits: A balanced dinner with lean protein and fiber-rich vegetables to keep you full and satisfied.

Day 12

Breakfast: Avocado and Egg Bowl

Ingredients:

•

2 eggs

•

1/2 avocado, diced

•

1/4 cup salsa (optional)

•

Salt and pepper to taste

Instructions:

1. Cook the eggs to your liking (fried or scrambled).

2. Serve over diced avocado, and top with salsa if desired.

3. Season with salt and pepper.

Benefits: This quick breakfast is loaded with healthy fats and protein, providing a great start to your day.

Lunch: Beef and Veggie Lettuce Wraps

Ingredients:

- 1/2 lb ground beef

- 1/4 onion, diced

- 1/2 bell pepper, diced

- 2 tablespoons coconut aminos

- 1 tablespoon olive oil

- 4-6 large lettuce leaves (for wraps)

Instructions:

1. Cook ground beef with onions and bell peppers in olive oil until browned.

2. Stir in coconut aminos and cook for 1-2 more minutes.

3. Serve the beef mixture in lettuce wraps.

Benefits: A low-carb, high-protein lunch with plenty of veggies and healthy fats.

Dinner: Zucchini Noodles with Meatballs

Ingredients:

- 4 oz ground turkey or beef

- 1/4 cup almond flour

- 1 egg

- 1 teaspoon garlic powder

- 1 tablespoon olive oil

-

2 zucchini, spiralized

-

1/2 cup marinara sauce (no added sugar)

Instructions:

1. Mix ground meat, almond flour, egg, and garlic powder. Form into meatballs.

2. Cook meatballs in olive oil until browned and cooked through.

3. Sauté zucchini noodles in olive oil for 2-3 minutes until tender.

4. Serve meatballs on top of zucchini noodles with marinara sauce.

Benefits: A grain-free alternative to pasta with protein-packed meatballs and fiber-rich zucchini noodles.

Day 13

Breakfast: Coconut Yogurt with Nuts and Seeds

Ingredients:

-

1/2 cup unsweetened coconut yogurt

-

1 tablespoon chia seeds

-

1 tablespoon pumpkin seeds

-

1 tablespoon almond butter

Instructions:

1. Scoop coconut yogurt into a bowl. 2. Top with chia seeds, pumpkin seeds, and almond butter.

Benefits: Packed with probiotics, healthy fats, and fiber, this breakfast is great for gut health.

Lunch: Chicken and Avocado Salad

Ingredients:

-

1 grilled chicken breast, sliced

-

2 cups mixed greens

-

1/2 avocado, sliced

-

1/4 cucumber, sliced

-

1 tablespoon olive oil

-

1 tablespoon apple cider vinegar

-

Salt and pepper to taste

Instructions:

1.

Toss mixed greens, cucumber, and avocado in a bowl.

2.

Top with grilled chicken and drizzle with olive oil and apple cider vinegar.

3.

Season with salt and pepper. Benefits: A protein-rich salad full of healthy fats and vitamins.

Dinner: Grilled Shrimp with Roasted Asparagus

-

Ingredients:

-

1/2 lb shrimp, peeled and deveined

-

1 bunch asparagus, trimmed

2 tablespoons olive oil

-

1 teaspoon garlic powder

-

Salt and pepper to taste

Instructions:

1. Grill shrimp until pink and cooked through.

2. Toss asparagus with olive oil, garlic powder, salt, and pepper. Roast at 400°F for 10-12 minutes.

3. Serve the shrimp with roasted asparagus.

Benefits: High in protein and rich in antioxidants, this meal supports your immune system and muscle recovery.

Day 14

Breakfast: Egg Muffins with Veggies

Ingredients:

- 4 eggs

- 1/4 cup spinach, chopped

- 1/4 cup bell pepper, diced

- 1 tablespoon olive oil

- Salt and pepper to taste

Instructions:

1. Preheat oven to 375°F (190°C).

2. Whisk eggs with salt and pepper, and stir in chopped vegetables.

3. Grease a muffin tin with olive oil and pour egg mixture into the cups. 4. Bake for 15-20 minutes until set.

Benefits: A portable, protein-rich breakfast with veggies for added fiber.

Lunch: Tuna Salad Lettuce Wraps

Ingredients:

-

1 can tuna, drained

-

1 tablespoon olive oil

-

1 tablespoon lemon juice

-

1/4 cucumber, diced

-

4 large lettuce leaves (for wraps)

Instructions:

1. Mix tuna with olive oil, lemon juice, and diced cucumber.

2. Serve the tuna mixture in lettuce wraps.

Benefits: A light and satisfying lunch high in protein and healthy fats.

Dinner: Baked Chicken Thighs with Roasted Carrots

Ingredients:

- 2 chicken thighs, bone-in, skin-on

- 2 cups carrots, sliced

- 2 tablespoons olive oil

- Salt and pepper to taste

Instructions:

1. Preheat the oven to 400°F (200°C).

2. Toss carrots with olive oil, salt, and pepper, and roast for 25-30 minutes.

3. Season chicken thighs with salt and pepper and bake for 35-40 minutes.

4. Serve with roasted carrots.

Benefits: A simple, hearty dinner with protein and fiber-rich vegetables.

Section 3: Dressings and Vinaigrettes

1. Lemon-Tahini Dressing

Ingredients:

-

1/4 cup tahini (sesame paste)

-

2 tablespoons fresh lemon juice

-

1 tablespoon olive oil

-

1 tablespoon water (to thin if needed)

-

1 small garlic clove, minced

-

1/2 teaspoon salt

-

1/4 teaspoon ground cumin (optional)

-

Fresh parsley, chopped (optional)

Instructions:

1. In a small bowl, whisk together the tahini, lemon juice, olive oil, garlic, and cumin.

2. Slowly add water to thin the dressing to your desired consistency.

3. Season with salt and garnish with chopped parsley if desired.

4. Use on salads, as a dip for veggies, or drizzled over roasted vegetables.

Benefits: This dressing is high in healthy fats, fiber, and minerals from tahini, with a boost of antioxidants from lemon.

2. Avocado-Cilantro Lime Dressing

Ingredients:

-

1 ripe avocado

•

2 tablespoons fresh lime juice

•

1/4 cup olive oil

•

1/4 cup water (or more, for desired consistency)

•

1/4 cup fresh cilantro, chopped

•

1 garlic clove

•

Salt and pepper to taste

Instructions:

1. Blend all ingredients in a food processor or blender until smooth and creamy.

•

2. Add more water if necessary to adjust the consistency.

3. Season

4. with salt and pepper to taste.

5. Serve over salads, grilled meats, or as a dip.

Benefits: This dressing is rich in healthy fats from avocado, which support skin, brain, and heart health, while cilantro adds a detoxifying boost.

3. Balsamic Vinaigrette

Ingredients:

1/4 cup balsamic vinegar (preferably aged)

•

1/2 cup extra virgin olive oil

•

1 teaspoon Dijon mustard

•

1 small garlic clove, minced

•

1 teaspoon honey (optional)

•

Salt and pepper to taste

Instructions:

1. Whisk together the balsamic vinegar, Dijon mustard, garlic, and honey (if using).

2. Slowly drizzle in the olive oil while whisking to emulsify.

3. Season with salt and pepper to taste.

4. Store in an airtight container in the refrigerator for up to a week.

Benefits: Balsamic vinegar is rich in antioxidants, and the olive oil adds heart-healthy fats. The mustard helps to create a creamy texture without using any dairy.

4. Coconut Cream Dressing

Ingredients:

- 1/4 cup coconut cream (from a can of coconut milk, refrigerated)

- 1 tablespoon apple cider vinegar

- 1 tablespoon fresh lemon juice

- 1 tablespoon olive oil

-

1 teaspoon Dijon mustard

-

1/4 teaspoon garlic powder

-

Salt and pepper to taste

Instructions:

1. Whisk together the coconut cream, apple cider vinegar, lemon juice, olive oil, Dijon 2. Add water if needed to thin the dressing to your preferred consistency.

3. Season with salt and pepper to taste.

4. Drizzle over salads, grilled vegetables, or roasted chicken.

Benefits: Coconut cream is full of healthy fats and lauric acid, which support immune health. This dressing provides a creamy texture without dairy.

5. Creamy Miso Dressing

Ingredients:

-

2 tablespoons white miso paste (look for grain-free miso)

*

2 tablespoons rice vinegar (or apple cider vinegar)

*

1 tablespoon sesame oil

*

1 tablespoon olive oil

*

1 tablespoon coconut aminos (optional, for sweetness)

*

1 teaspoon grated ginger

*

1 garlic clove, minced

Instructions:

1. Whisk together the miso paste, vinegar, sesame oil, olive oil, coconut aminos, ginger, and garlic.

2. Add water to thin, if necessary, until the dressing is smooth and pourable.

3. Drizzle over salads, steamed veggies, or grilled fish.

Benefits: Miso provides probiotics for gut health, while sesame oil adds a rich, nutty flavor and antiinflammatory properties.

6. Herb and Garlic Pesto

Ingredients:

-

1 cup fresh basil leaves (or a mix of basil, parsley, and cilantro)

-

1/4 cup pine nuts (or walnuts)

-

2 garlic cloves

-

1/4 cup olive oil

-

1/4 cup Parmesan cheese (optional, or nutritional yeast for dairy-free)

-

Salt and pepper to taste

-

1 tablespoon lemon juice (optional)

Instructions:

1. In a food processor, combine the herbs, pine nuts, and garlic. Pulse until finely chopped.

2. Slowly drizzle in olive oil while processing until the pesto reaches your desired consistency.

3. Stir in Parmesan cheese (or nutritional yeast) and season with salt, pepper, and lemon juice.

4. Use as a dressing, a sauce for meats or vegetables, or a topping for roasted vegetables.

Benefits: Full of fresh herbs, garlic, and healthy fats, this pesto is rich in antioxidants, vitamins, and hearthealthy fats.

7. Spicy Mustard Vinaigrette

Ingredients:

•

2 tablespoons Dijon mustard

•

2 tablespoons apple cider vinegar

•

1/4 cup olive oil

-

1/4 teaspoon smoked paprika (optional for smoky flavor)

-

1/4 teaspoon cayenne pepper (optional for heat)

-

Salt and pepper to taste

Instructions:

1. Whisk together the Dijon mustard, apple cider vinegar, smoked paprika, and cayenne pepper.

2. Slowly drizzle in olive oil while whisking to emulsify.

-

3. Season with salt and pepper to taste. 4. Perfect for drizzling over salads, roasted veggies, or grilled meats.

Benefits: Mustard provides a sharp, tangy flavor with no added sugars, while apple cider vinegar offers digestive benefits and anti-inflammatory properties.

These dressings and sauces can be used on salads, roasted veggies, grilled meats, or as dips for raw vegetables. They are all made from nutrient-dense ingredients and will help add variety and flavor to meals while staying true to the Savage Diet principles.

Section 4: Teas

1. Ginger-Lemon Detox Tea

Ingredients:

•

1-inch piece of fresh ginger, peeled and thinly sliced

•

1/2 lemon, sliced

•

1 teaspoon honey (optional, for sweetness)

•

2 cups hot water

A pinch of cayenne pepper (optional, for an extra kick)

Instructions:

1. Bring 2 cups of water to a boil.

2. Add the sliced ginger and let it simmer for 5–10 minutes. The longer it simmers, the stronger the ginger flavor will be.

3. Add the lemon slices and simmer for an additional 2–3 minutes.

4. Strain the tea into a cup.

5. Stir in honey if desired, and a pinch of cayenne pepper if you want an extra zing.

6. Enjoy while it's warm.

Benefits: This tea is great for digestion and detoxification. Ginger is known for its anti-inflammatory properties, while lemon provides a boost of vitamin C. Cayenne pepper can help stimulate metabolism.

2. Chamomile-Lavender Relaxation Tea

Ingredients:

•

1 tablespoon dried chamomile flowers

•

1 tablespoon dried lavender flowers

•

1–2 teaspoons honey (optional, for sweetness)

•

2 cups hot water

Instructions:

1. Boil 2 cups of water.

2. Place the chamomile and lavender flowers in a tea infuser or directly into your teapot.

3. Pour the hot water over the flowers and steep for 5–7 minutes, depending on how strong you want the flavor.

4. Strain the tea into a cup.

5. Sweeten with honey if desired.

6. Sip slowly and relax.

Benefits: Chamomile and lavender are both well-known for their calming properties. This tea is perfect for winding down at night, reducing stress, and promoting restful sleep.

3. Mint and Lemon Balm Digestive Tea

Ingredients:

-

1 tablespoon fresh mint leaves (or 1 teaspoon dried mint)

-

1 tablespoon fresh lemon balm leaves (or 1 teaspoon dried lemon balm)

-

1 teaspoon honey (optional, for sweetness)

•

2 cups hot water

Instructions:

1. Boil 2 cups of water.

2. Add the fresh mint and lemon balm leaves to a teapot or mug.

3. Pour the hot water over the herbs and let steep for 5–7 minutes.

4. Strain the tea into a cup.

5. Sweeten with honey if desired.

6. Drink this tea after meals to help with digestion.

Benefits: Mint and lemon balm are excellent for soothing the digestive system, easing bloating, and promoting healthy digestion. This tea is ideal for settling your stomach after a meal.

•

1. Turmeric-Ginger Immune Boost Tea

Ingredients:

-

1-inch piece of fresh ginger, peeled and sliced

-

1/2 teaspoon ground turmeric (or 1-inch fresh turmeric root, peeled and sliced)

-

1/2 lemon, juiced

-

1 teaspoon honey (optional, for sweetness)

-

2 cups hot water

-

Pinch of black pepper (helps with turmeric absorption)

Instructions:

1. Bring 2 cups of water to a boil.

2. Add the ginger and turmeric slices to the water, and simmer for 5–10 minutes.

3. Remove from heat and strain the tea into a cup.

4. Stir in lemon juice, honey, and a pinch of black pepper.

5. Drink while warm for maximum benefits.

Benefits: Turmeric and ginger are both anti-inflammatory and immune-boosting, while lemon adds vitamin C, and black pepper helps improve the absorption of curcumin (the active ingredient in turmeric).

2. Lemon Balm and Peppermint Tea

Ingredients:

•

1 tablespoon fresh lemon balm leaves (or 1 teaspoon dried)

•

1 tablespoon fresh peppermint leaves (or 1 teaspoon dried)

•

2 cups hot water

•

1 teaspoon honey (optional, for sweetness)

Instructions:

1. Boil 2 cups of water.

2. Add the lemon balm and peppermint leaves to a tea infuser or directly into the teapot.

3. Pour the hot water over the herbs and steep for 5–7 minutes.

4. Strain the tea into a cup and sweeten with honey if desired.

5. Enjoy warm or iced.

Benefits: Lemon balm and peppermint both have calming effects, making this tea perfect for relieving stress and soothing digestive discomfort. It's also great for enhancing mental clarity and reducing anxiety.

3. Cinnamon-Apple Spice Tea

Ingredients:

•

1 cinnamon stick

•

2 slices of fresh apple (or 1/4 cup apple slices, dried)

•

2–3 whole cloves

•

2 cups hot water

•

1 teaspoon honey (optional)

Instructions:

1. Boil 2 cups of water in a small saucepan.

2. Add the cinnamon stick, apple slices, and cloves to the water.

3. Let the mixture simmer for about 10–15 minutes for a strong, aromatic flavor.

4. Strain the tea into a cup, and stir in honey if desired.

5. Serve hot for a warming and comforting drink.

Benefits: This tea has a warming, comforting flavor, thanks to the cinnamon and apple. Cinnamon is great for stabilizing blood sugar levels, and cloves offer antioxidant and anti-inflammatory benefits.

Section 5: Healthy Snacks

Healthy Snack 1: Nut and Seed Energy Bars

Ingredients:

•

1/4 cup almonds

•

1/4 cup walnuts

•

1/4 cup sunflower seeds

•

1/4 cup pumpkin seeds

•

1 tablespoon chia seeds

•

1 tablespoon coconut oil

•

1 tablespoon raw honey

•

1/4 teaspoon vanilla extract

Instructions:

1. Pulse the almonds, walnuts, and seeds in a food processor until chopped but not fully ground.

2. In a small saucepan, melt the coconut oil and honey over low heat.

3. Stir in the vanilla extract.

4. Mix the wet ingredients with the chopped nuts and seeds and press the mixture into a parchmentlined pan.

5. Refrigerate for an hour, then cut into bars.

Benefits: This snack is loaded with healthy fats, protein, and fiber to keep you full between meals and support energy levels throughout the day.

Healthy Snack 2: Veggie and Hummus Dip

Ingredients:

-

1/2 cup carrot sticks

-

1/2 cup cucumber slices

-

1/2 cup celery sticks

-

1/4 cup homemade or store-bought hummus (grain-free)

Instructions:

1. Slice your veggies into sticks.

2. Serve with a side of hummus for dipping.

Benefits: Low-calorie, high-fiber snack that's rich in vitamins and antioxidants from the fresh vegetables.

Hummus provides protein and healthy fats.

Snack 3: Cucumber and Hummus

Ingredients:

- 1/2 cucumber, sliced

- 1/4 cup homemade or store-bought hummus (grain-free)

Instructions:

1. Slice the cucumber and serve with hummus for dipping.

Benefits: A refreshing and hydrating snack with healthy fats and fiber.

Snack 4: Walnuts and Berries

Ingredients:

-

1/4 cup walnuts

-

1/2 cup mixed berries (such as blueberries, raspberries, and blackberries) Instructions: 1. Combine walnuts and berries for a nutrient-dense snack.

Benefits: Packed with antioxidants and omega-3 fatty acids, this snack promotes brain health and energy.

Snack 5: Celery with Almond Butter

Ingredients:

-

2-3 celery sticks

-

2 tablespoons almond butter

Instructions:

1. Spread almond butter on celery sticks for a satisfying snack.

Benefits: Rich in healthy fats and fiber, this snack supports satiety and energy.

Snack 6: Hard-Boiled Eggs

Ingredients:

-

2 hard-boiled eggs

Instructions: 1. Boil eggs, peel them, and enjoy for a quick, high-protein snack.

Benefits: A simple, protein-packed snack that supports muscle recovery and energy.

Snack 7: Coconut and Almond Energy Balls

Ingredients:

-

1/4 cup unsweetened shredded coconut

-

1/4 cup almonds, chopped

-

1 tablespoon almond butter

-

1 tablespoon honey or maple syrup

-

1 tablespoon chia seeds

Instructions:

1. In a bowl, mix all ingredients together until well combined.

2. Roll the mixture into small balls and refrigerate for at least 30 minutes.

Benefits: A healthy, nutrient-dense snack with healthy fats, fiber, and a natural energy boost.

Snack 8: Cucumber and Guacamole

Ingredients:

-

1/2 cucumber, sliced

-

1/4 cup guacamole (homemade or store-bought)

Instructions:

1. Slice cucumber into rounds and serve with guacamole for dipping.

Benefits: A light, hydrating snack packed with healthy fats and antioxidants.

Snack 9: Almonds and Dried Apricots

Ingredients:

-

1/4 cup almonds

-

2-3 dried apricots (unsweetened)

Instructions:

1. Enjoy almonds and dried apricots for a sweet and salty snack.

Benefits: A satisfying mix of healthy fats, fiber, and natural sugars to fuel your day.

Snack 10: Veggie Sticks with Tahini Dip

Ingredients:

-

1/2 cup celery sticks

-

1/2 cup carrot sticks

-

2 tablespoons tahini

Instructions: 1. Dip veggie sticks into tahini for a rich, creamy, nutrient-dense snack.

Benefits: High in fiber and healthy fats, this snack supports digestion and provides a natural energy boost.

Snack 11: Walnuts and Goji Berries

Ingredients:

-

1/4 cup walnuts

-

2 tablespoons goji berries (dried, unsweetened)

Instructions: 1. Combine walnuts and goji berries for a nutrient-packed snack.

Benefits: A great source of antioxidants and healthy fats to support skin health and energy.

Snack 12: Hard-Boiled Eggs with Pickles

Ingredients:

-

2 hard-boiled eggs

-

2-3 dill pickles (fermented)

Instructions:

1. Pair hard-boiled eggs with fermented pickles for a high-protein, gut-friendly Snack 13: Cucumber and Avocado Dip

Ingredients:

- 1/2 cucumber, peeled and chopped

- 1/2 avocado, peeled and pitted

- 1 tablespoon fresh lemon juice

- 1 tablespoon olive oil

- Salt and pepper to taste

Instructions:

1. Mash the avocado in a bowl, then add the chopped cucumber, lemon juice, and olive oil.

2. Stir to combine, and season with salt and pepper.

3. Serve as a refreshing dip with veggie sticks or as a snack on its own.

Benefits: This dip is hydrating and full of healthy fats from avocado and olive oil, making it a great light snack.

Snack 14: Mixed Nuts and Berries

Ingredients:

-

1/4 cup mixed nuts (such as almonds, walnuts, and pecans)

-

1/4 cup mixed berries (blueberries, raspberries, or strawberries)
Instructions:

1. Combine the nuts and berries in a small bowl or snack container. 2.

Enjoy as a satisfying, nutrient-packed snack.

Benefits: A simple, nutrient-dense snack with healthy fats, fiber, and antioxidants from the berries and nuts.

Part IV: The Lifestyle of the Modern Savage

Chapter 9: Living the Active Ancestral Life

The air felt different today, charged with a stillness that sent ripples of unease through the bones of my people. The canyon walls, steep and unyielding, rose around us like ancient sentinels, their jagged peaks cutting into the sky. The path was narrow, winding between massive boulders, yet it felt familiar, like the steady pulse of the earth beneath our feet. Our tribe moved with practiced grace, each step measured, aware of the narrow path ahead.

But today, something was wrong. The wind had shifted, moving in sharp, erratic bursts, carrying a chill that none of us had expected. I felt it first on the back of my neck, a cold breeze whispering promises of something unseen, something dangerous. We had traveled through canyons like this before, though never with the heavy, ominous clouds that now hung low in the sky. The sky, once a clear expanse of blue, had turned dark—a bruise against the horizon. It was no longer the gentle transition from day to evening; this felt different, violent, almost like the earth itself was breathing in slow, deep inhales, preparing to strike.

I glanced back at my people—our elders, our children, our hunters—moving with the same quiet resolve we always carried, but there was a subtle tension in their movements. Even the youngest felt it, a primal instinct gnawing at the edges of their thoughts, just as it gnawed at mine.

It was then that I heard it—a rumble deep in the earth. Not a sound, but a vibration, something you feel before you hear. My heart raced, and I turned to the elder who walked beside me, Naka, her face weathered by age, yet always sharp with insight. She looked at me, eyes narrowed. "We need to move faster," she said, her voice a low, urgent whisper.

I nodded, pulling my spear closer. The hunters were already preparing, their eyes scanning the rock faces and distant ridgelines. They could sense it too. Something was coming.

And then, it arrived. The wind shifted once again, this time with the force of a storm. The sky, once a deep gray, turned black—swirling clouds churning like a massive beast stirring from its slumber. A torrent of rain, thick and sudden, poured from the heavens, washing over us in an instant. The sound was deafening, the wind howling so loud that even our warriors could barely hear each other over its fury.

Lightning cracked through the dark sky, illuminating the jagged rock faces and casting fleeting shadows that twisted and writhed like the spirits of the dead. In the chaos of the storm, we saw them.

At first, they were mere shapes, silhouettes against the violent backdrop of the canyon. Then, as the lightning illuminated the land, they became clear—massive, towering creatures, their bodies thick with muscle and power. Mammoths—were beasts of ancient size, more dangerous than anything we had seen in a long time.

I spotted one immediately—its enormous frame moving with the precision of a predator, the ground trembling beneath its weight. A mammoth. But not just any mammoth—this one was enormous, its tusks curving dangerously, sweeping the air like great weapons. Behind it, I saw the unmistakable outline of a saber-toothed tiger, its teeth bared in a silent roar, moving toward us with deadly intent. Their size, their power—it was like the earth itself had decided to challenge our existence.

"Move!" I shouted, my voice barely audible over the storm's fury. "Move, now!" Panic swept through the tribe as the realization hit. We had to cross the canyon's narrow pass quickly or be trapped between the storm and the charging beasts. I turned to Naka, who had already begun to shout commands to the elders, guiding them with her calm, unwavering authority. We had prepared for many dangers in our lives—droughts, predators, the fierce elements—but nothing like this. The storm had come without

warning, and the megafauna, disturbed by the change in the weather, were coming toward us like a wall of unstoppable force.

I motioned to the hunters, who immediately split off, each one moving with speed and purpose, their spears and arrows ready. Our weapons were no match for the size of the beasts, but we would need to distract them, to buy time for the children and elders to escape.

The mammoth charged first, its massive feet pounding against the earth, shaking the canyon floor. I could feel the vibrations deep in my chest. Its tusks gleamed in the dim light, aiming directly at the path our tribe had taken. I drew my spear, feeling the weight of it in my hand as I readied myself. But it was too late for hesitation. The ground beneath me shifted—rocks and earth cracking as the storm raged on. The mammoth roared, its enormous body moving with terrifying speed, and I knew in that moment that we were facing something beyond even our greatest challenges. We would either face it with the strength of our ancestors or perish, like the many before us who had not been strong enough.

The roar of the storm and the pounding of the large beasts were deafening now. I looked around, seeing the fear in the eyes of my people—but there was no time for fear, only action. With a deep breath, I motioned to the others, signaling that we must not turn back. Together, we would face this storm.

Together, we would fight for our survival. The earth trembled beneath us, and the battle for our very lives had only just begun.

Section 1: The Physical Savage Life

The focus on the Savage lifestyle should be movements that connect us with not only our earth but also of functionality and the ability to mimic our ancestor's way of movement. For example, in gathering the greens that they did on a daily basis, they moved, whether through squatting, crawling, lifting or sprinting.

They had to crawl up the sides of hills and boulders, they bent over reaching, and possibly at times had to crawl. These movements, I believe, were not only essential for building strength, but also for enhancing mobility and agility.

Our ancestors engaged their whole body in their movements. I am sure they didn't look at their bicep and go, "I need to do a little more bicep curls". But on a daily basis they used their biceps, and they engaged multiple muscle groups, that on the whole, promoted overall functional fitness.

The foods that are included in The Savage Diet, are rich in protein, healthy fats, and whole foods. They naturally supply the energy and nutrients that are needed for effective physical movement. When you use the right fuel, this enhances muscle recovery, and boosts endurance, promotes fat loss, which as a Savage, will help you endure the cold climate and be able to hunt and fight off the scary Saber-tooth tiger.

It also promotes fat loss, which is essential for sustained performance in any physical activity. By naturally eliminating processed grains and sugars, the body is more able to rely on fats for energy, which is ideal for endurance-based activities, such as walking for long distances searching for food or quick sprinting movements necessary to kill the Saber-toothed tiger or elk.

I believe that incorporating Animal Flow exercises that mimic animal movements, such as the bear crawl, crab reach, and ape jumps will help promote mobility, flexibility and strength while being in tune with nature.

A Primal Circuit workout that combines movements like pushing, pulling, lifting, jumping, crawling, and running are workouts that mimic how our ancestors might have interacted with their environment, improving full-body strength, agility and cardiovascular health.

Section 2: Flexibility, Mobility and Stability

The importance of joint health cannot be understated. I will always encourage exercises that improve flexibility and joint health, which to me are key for long-term functional fitness. As we age, we are not thinking about "Oh I can't do this exercise anymore". We always try to do it, even cartwheels, until we see we can't do it. But it is too late by then, and we have sprained or broken something. This is why I tell each of my patients we have to get a bone density done before we start on a program, so I can see where we are starting from. You have to keep your bones healthy. The way to do this, is not by taking a pill or a an injection, that you are told will help rebuild your bones. In all honesty, your body is not deficient in a pill. It is deficient in movement, it is deficient in certain supplements, such as Vitamin D, calcium, Zinc, Copper, Manganese, and Vitamin K, and walking in a purposeful manner. Practices such as deep squats, lunges and dynamic stretches are great for opening up the hips, improving posture and increasing mobility. I need to stress that a strong core, not just for strength, but for injury prevention, and overall balance needs to be a part of your physical program. If you fall, your body has to be strong enough to protect you from fracturing "the proverbial hip". These are not easy, and you will have to work up to them. I do not place any time frame on them, I want you to try, every day, just try. Do a little more each time you work out, and pretty soon, you will have them down where they are not difficult to do.

There is also a Vibrational plate to be set at the setting for building bone matrix, this does help for keeping osteoporosis at bay, as long as you do all the other things such as intentional walking, hiking and eating a good, clean diet such as the Savage Diet.

This exercise program is not hard to do, but you have to practice the part where you just show every day.

Start with planks, leg raises, and plain windmills. Look on YouTube or go to www.thesavagediet.com if you need help with the movement.

Mindful Movement

I suggest incorporating yoga and other mobility-focused practices such as Tai Chi, or QiGong to balance out strength training. This will help improve the mind-body connection, flexibility, and breath control.

Outdoors

This is my favorite. I always try to encourage physical activity in the outdoors. Choosing natural environments like parks, forests or hiking trails. Try to walk or run (a little) on varied terrain is much more beneficial for the body than on a flat surface, it engages more muscles and it improves your balance. You can start incorporating functional training tools by using objects like rocks, logs, sandbags, kettlebells or tire flips for a more rugged or primal form of strength training.

Doing sprints or hill climbs with short, intense bursts of activity followed by periods of rest (similar to HIIT) mimics the bursts of energy needed in real-life situations- such as sprinting after prey or quickly escaping danger. I encourage exercises (if you are in good shape) that focus on explosive power, like jumping over obstacles or climbing ropes, which engage the whole body and improve agility.

Another activity I enjoy is orienteering. It typically takes place outdoors, and you can participate alone, with a partner, or in a team as you navigate a map to designated locations and mark each one off. The first team to arrive wins. However, if you can't locate all the sites and miss one, you'll just end up getting a lot of exercise.

Section 3: Total-Body Workouts for Sustainability

Full-body workouts engage the body holistically and are excellent for building strength without the need for complex machines or weights. So, you can do movements like squats, lunges, push-ups, pull-ups, and deadlifts to engage the body. Keep the workout program simple, requiring minimal to no equipment.

Bodyweight exercises, outdoor running, swimming, or cycling should be at the forefront, with the focus on functional and practical fitness rather than gym-specific movements.

Movement As a Lifestyle

I would like you to be aware of your movements throughout the day. Beyond any structured workouts, stay active, for example, if you have to go shopping, park further away from the door, and walk to your car. Use the stairs instead of the elevator, and try a recreational activity like Pickleball or Sports dancing.

Remember to rest also. Do not think that our ancestors were out working all day, they rested too. Just as the body needs nutrient-dense foods from the Savage Diet, it also requires adequate sleep and recovery to repair muscles and prevent overtraining.

Section 4: Savage Lifestyle Physical Exercise Program

The frequency should be: 3-4 times a week (with rest days for recovery) Always do this first: Warm-Up (5-10 minutes)

•

Dynamic Stretching (Arm circles, leg swings, hip circles)

-

Joint Mobility (Neck, shoulders, wrists, hips, knees, and ankles)

-

Light Cardio (Jumping jacks, light jogging, or cycling)

Workout Structure

This program follows a circuit-style format, incorporating different movement patterns to work the entire body. Each day we will focus on a mix of strength, mobility, endurance, and functional movement. Perform each exercise for 30-45 seconds, and over time increase to 60 seconds, followed by 15-30 seconds of rest between exercises.

After completing all exercises, rest for 1-2 minutes, then repeat the circuit for 3-4 rounds.

Day 1: Full-Body Strength and Mobility Focus

1. Animal Flow: Beast Crawl

-

Crawl on all fours with knees off the ground. Focus on smooth, controlled movements. • This will benefit: Full-body engagement, core stability, and mobility.

2. Primal Push-Ups with Shoulder Taps • Perform a push-up, then at the top, tap each shoulder with the opposite hand for added core stability.

•

This will benefit: Upper body strength, core stability.

3. Goblet Squats (using a kettlebell or dumbbell)

•

Hold a weight in front of you and squat deeply, keeping your chest upright.

•

This will benefit: Lower body strength, flexibility, and mobility.

4. Lateral Lunges

•

Step to the side and squat down with one leg, keeping the other leg straight.

•

This will benefit: Strengthen hips, glutes, and quads while enhancing lateral mobility.

5. Plank with Reach

•

In a plank position, alternate reaching one arm forward while maintaining stability with the other.

-

This will benefit: Core strength and stability.

6. Cat-Cow Stretch

-

On all fours, alternate between arching your back (cow) and rounding it (cat).

-

This will benefit: Spinal mobility, flexibility, and posture improvement.

Day 2: Functional Strength and Endurance Focus

1. Kettlebell Swings

-

Swing the kettlebell between your legs and up to shoulder height, using your hips to generate the movement.

-

This will benefit: Hip power, posterior chain development, and cardiovascular conditioning.

2. Bear Crawl

-

Crawl forward on all fours, keeping your knees off the ground and your core engaged. • This will benefit: Full-body movement, core strength, and shoulder stability.

3. Jump Squats

-

Perform a squat, then explode upward into a jump. Land softly back into a squat.

-

This will benefit: Leg power, explosiveness, and cardiovascular fitness.

4. Burpees

-

Perform a squat thrust into a push-up, then jump explosively into the air. • This will benefit: Full-body workout, it will improve cardiovascular fitness and strength.

5. Mountain Climbers • Start in a plank position and alternate bringing your knees towards your chest quickly, as if you're running in place.

-

It will benefit: Core activation, cardiovascular conditioning.

6. Deep Squat Hold

-

Lower into a deep squat and hold for 30-60 seconds.

-

It will benefit: Mobility and flexibility in the hips, ankles, and lower back.

Day 3: Core Stability, Agility, and Mobility Focus

1. Dead Bugs

-

Lie on your back, extend one leg straight while lowering the opposite arm towards the floor, then return to starting position and alternate.

-

This will benefit: Core stabilization, coordination.

2. Side Plank with Leg Raises

-

From a side plank position, raise your top leg while maintaining balance.

-

Benefit: Strengthen the obliques, shoulders, and hips.

3. Single-Leg Deadlifts (Bodyweight or Kettlebell) • Balance on one leg, hinge at the hips, and lower the weight (or just your body) toward the ground before returning to standing.

-

This will benefit: Hamstring and glute strength, balance.

4. Box Jumps (or Vertical Jumps)

-

Jump onto a stable box or platform (or perform vertical jumps if no box is available).

-

This will benefit: Explosive power and leg strength.

5. Bear Crawl to Crab Reach • Start in a bear crawl position, then rotate into a crab position, reaching one arm overhead to stretch the chest. •

This will benefit: Mobility, shoulder stability, and full-body coordination.

6. Thoracic Spine Rotation

-

Sit or kneel, rotate your torso and reach one arm overhead, stretching the thoracic spine.

-

This will benefit: Upper back and thoracic spine mobility, improves posture.

Day 4: Agility, Strength, and Outdoor Focus

1. Sprints (or Hill Climbs)

-

Sprint for 20-30 seconds, then rest for 1 minute.

-

This will benefit: Explosive cardiovascular conditioning, leg strength.

2. Lunge Jumps

-

Jump into a lunge position, then explode into the air and switch legs mid-flight.

-

This will benefit: Leg power, explosiveness, and endurance.

3. Farmer's Walk (Using Dumbbells or Kettlebells)

-

Hold a heavy weight in each hand and walk for a set distance or time. • This will benefit: Full-body strength, grip strength, and endurance.

4. Tire Flips (if available)

-

Flip a large tire or use a heavy object to mimic the motion. •

This will benefit: Full-body

strength, explosive power.

5. Climbing or Rope Pulls (if available)

-

If you can access a rope or climbing structure, work on climbing or pulling yourself up.

-

This will benefit: Upper body strength, grip strength, and endurance.

6. Walking Lunges with Rotation

-

Lunge forward and twist your torso over the front leg, engaging the core.

-

This will benefit: Core stability, mobility, and leg strength.

Cool Down (5-10 minutes):

-

Stretching: Focus on stretching the hip flexors, hamstrings, quads, shoulders, and lower back.

-

Breathing exercises: Deep diaphragmatic breathing to aid in relaxation and recovery.

-

Intensity: Gradually increase the intensity by adding more rounds, increasing the time per exercise, or using heavier resistance (kettlebells, sandbags).

-

Rest: Rest for 1-2 minutes between rounds, and take active rest (walking or light movement) if necessary.

-

Frequency: Perform this program 3-4 times per week with active recovery or rest days in between (e.g., yoga, stretching, or walking).

Savage Lifestyle Physical Exercise Program: Expanded

Frequency: 3-4 times per week

Warm-Up (5-10 minutes):

-

Joint Mobility: Neck, shoulders, wrists, hips, knees, and ankles.

-

Dynamic Stretching: Arm circles, leg swings, hip openers.

-

Light Cardio: Jump rope, jogging, high knees, or butt kicks.

Workout Structure (Circuit-Style)

Perform each exercise for 30-45 seconds, and over time increase to 60 seconds, followed by 15-30

seconds of rest between exercises. After completing all exercises, rest for 1-2 minutes, then repeat the circuit for 3-4 rounds.

Day 1: Full-Body Strength & Mobility Focus

1. Animal Flow: Beast Crawl (Option 1) •

Crawl on all fours, keeping your knees off the ground

and moving forward. Can alternate with a Crab Crawl for variety. •

This will benefit: Full-body

engagement, core stability, and mobility.

2. Primal Push-Ups with Shoulder Taps (Option 2) •

Perform a push-up, then tap each shoulder at

the top. You can also add a Clapping Push-Up for an explosive challenge.

•

This will benefit: Upper body strength, core stability.

3. Goblet Squats with Kettlebell (Option 1)

•

Hold a kettlebell or dumbbell in front of your chest and perform deep squats. Try Overhead Squats for more intensity.

-

This will benefit: Lower body strength, flexibility, and mobility.

4. Lateral Lunges (Option 2) • Step to the side and squat down with one leg, keeping the other leg straight. You can modify this by adding a Lateral Lunge Jump for more intensity. •

This will

benefit: Strengthens hips, glutes, and quads while enhancing lateral mobility.

5. Plank with Reach (Option 3) •

In a plank position, alternate reaching one arm forward while maintaining stability with the other.

You can also do a Side Plank with Leg Lift for variety.

-

This will benefit: Core strength and stability.

6. Cat-Cow Stretch (Option 4) • On all fours, alternate between arching your back (cow) and rounding it (cat). For a deeper stretch, try Thread the Needle.

-

This will benefit: Spinal mobility, flexibility, and posture improvement.

Day 2: Functional Strength & Endurance Focus

1. Kettlebell Swings (Option 1) • Perform a kettlebell swing, thrusting the hips forward to engage the posterior chain. You can switch to Russian Swings for a higher arc.

•

This will benefit: Hip power, posterior chain development, and cardiovascular conditioning.

2. Bear Crawl (Option 2)

•

Crawl on all fours, keeping your knees off the ground. Add a Bear Crawl to Crab Reach for a dynamic movement challenge. •

This will benefit: Full-body movement, core strength, and

shoulder stability.

3. Jump Squats (Option 3) •

Perform a squat, then explode upward into a jump. Modify with Split Squat Jumps for unilateral leg strength.

•

This will benefit: Leg power, explosiveness, and cardiovascular fitness.

4. Burpees (Option 4) • Perform a squat thrust into a push-up, then jump explosively. For an extra challenge, try Burpee Broad Jumps. • This will benefit: Full-body workout, improves cardiovascular fitness and strength.

5. Mountain Climbers (Option 5)

•

In a plank position, alternate bringing your knees towards your chest quickly, as if you're running in place. Cross-body mountain climbers are an excellent variation for more core engagement.

•

This will benefit: Core activation, cardiovascular conditioning.

6. Deep Squat Hold (Option 6) •

Hold a deep squat position, focusing on posture and

breathing. You can try Goblet Squat Holds for added resistance.

•

This will benefit: Mobility and flexibility in the hips, ankles, and lower back.

Day 3: Core Stability, Agility & Mobility Focus

1. Dead Bugs (Option 1)

•

Lie on your back, extend one leg straight while lowering the opposite arm toward the floor, then return to starting position and alternate. Try Dead Bugs with a Stability Ball for extra core engagement.

•

This will benefit: Core stabilization, coordination.

2. Side Plank with Leg Raises (Option 2) •

From a side plank position, raise your top leg while

maintaining balance. Side Plank with Hip Dips is an alternative for targeting obliques.

•

This will benefit: Strengthen the obliques, shoulders, and hips.

3. Single-Leg Deadlifts (Bodyweight or Kettlebell) (Option 3) •

Balance on one leg, hinge at the hips,

and lower the weight (or just your body) toward the ground before returning to standing. You can use Resistance Bands for added difficulty.

•

This will benefit: Hamstring and glute strength, balance.

4. Box Jumps (or Vertical Jumps) (Option 4) • Jump onto a stable box or platform (or perform vertical jumps if no box is available). Try Depth Jumps for a more explosive version.

•

This will benefit: Explosive power and leg strength.

5. Bear Crawl to Crab Reach (Option 5)

•

Start in a bear crawl position, then rotate into a crab position, reaching one arm overhead to stretch the chest. You can alternate with a Crawl-to-Push-Up. • This will benefit: Mobility, shoulder stability, and full-body coordination.

6. Thoracic Spine Rotation (Option 6)

•

Sit or kneel, rotate your torso and reach one arm overhead, stretching the thoracic spine. For more of a challenge, try Thoracic Spine Rotations with a Band.

•

This will benefit: Upper back and thoracic spine mobility, improves posture.

Day 4: Agility, Strength & Outdoor Focus

1. Sprints (Option 1) • Sprint for 20-30 seconds, then rest for 1 minute. You can modify this with Hill Sprints for an increased challenge. • This will benefit: Explosive cardiovascular conditioning, leg strength.

2. Lunge Jumps (Option 2) •

Jump into a lunge position, then explode into the air and switch legs mid-flight. Try Bulgarian Split Squat Jumps for a more intense focus on one leg at a time.

•

This will benefit: Leg power, explosiveness, and endurance.

3. Farmer's Walk (Option 3) • Hold a heavy weight in each hand and walk for a set distance or time.

You can also try Overhead Farmer's Walks to challenge your shoulders and core. •

This will

benefit: Full-body strength, grip strength, and endurance.

4. Tire Flips (Option 4)

•

Flip a large tire or use a heavy object to mimic the motion. Another alternative is Sledgehammer Swings for a full-body workout. •

This will benefit: Full-body strength, explosive power.

. Climbing or Rope Pulls (Option 5)

•

If you have access to a rope or climbing structure, work on climbing or pulling yourself up. Rope Climbs are an excellent full-body challenge.

•

This will benefit: Upper body strength, grip strength, and endurance.

6. Walking Lunges with Rotation (Option 6) •

Lunge forward and twist your torso over the front leg,

engaging the core. Lunge with Overhead Reach is a great variation for added mobility.

•

This will benefit: Core stability, mobility, and leg strength.

Cool Down (5-10 minutes):

•

Stretching: Focus on stretching the hip flexors, hamstrings, quads, shoulders, and lower back.

-

Breathing exercises: Deep diaphragmatic breathing to aid in relaxation and recovery.

Progression Options:

-

Intensity: Gradually increase the intensity by adding more rounds, increasing the time per exercise, or using heavier resistance (kettlebells, sandbags).

-

Rest: Rest for 1-2 minutes between rounds, and take active rest (walking or light movement) if necessary.

-

Frequency: Perform this program 3-4 times per week with active recovery or rest days in between (e.g., yoga, stretching, or walking).

Part V: Navigating Modern Medicine as A Savage

Chapter 10: The Savage Diet and Medicine

Section 1: The Role of Diet in Disease Prevention and Management In a world that has embraced the convenience and speed of modern medicine, there is often little room for the timeless wisdom of the human body's natural healing abilities. Yet, as we embrace The Savage Diet and ancestral ways of living, it becomes increasingly clear that our journey is one of integration –

understanding how to navigate modern medicine while staying true to the ancient principles that have sustained us for millions of years.

Modern medicine has brought significant advancements that save lives, relieve suffering and offer a level of care that, in many ways, was once unimaginable. From antibiotics that fight infection to cutting-edge surgeries that repair and restore, these advancements have undoubtedly played a vital role in improving human health and longevity. But, as with everything in life, there is a balance. We must not surrender our autonomy over our bodies to these systems, but instead learn how to use them wisely – while still honoring the ancient wisdom of our bodies, mind, and spirit.

Section 2: Understanding the Divide: Ancestral Healing vs. Modern Medicine.

For tens of thousands of years our ancestors relied on nature for healing. They used herbs, foods, physical movement, and spiritual practices to prevent and address illness. The body was viewed as a holistic entity – each part deeply interconnected with the others – and the goal was always to restore balance. The foundation of this approach lies in what we now know as bioharmony, a principle that emphasizes the body's natural ability to heal itself when given the right tools.

In contrast, modern medicine has been designed with a focus on symptom treatment. While this is important in addressing immediate issues, it often overlooks root causes of health problems. The use of pharmaceuticals, invasive procedures and technologies can sometimes provide short-term solutions, but they rarely address the underlying imbalances in the body that can lead to chronic diseases.

This isn't to say that modern medicine is without merit – far from it. The key lies in understanding when to embrace the tools of modern science and when to turn to the ancestral knowledge that has stood the test of time. It is important to have a balance between the medicines and the modalities they both offer.

Section 3: When to Turn to Modern Medicine

There are times in life when the body requires outside intervention, and modern medicine provides solutions that our ancestors could not have dreamed of. Acute injuries, infections, and life-threatening conditions such as heart-attacks, strokes or accidents are situations where modern medicine is indispensable. For example, if you are involved in a serious car accident and experience trauma, you need immediate medical attention. Surgery, stitches, and intensive care can save your life, similarly, in the case of bacterial infections. Antibiotics can be a life-saving treatment that prevents the spread of harmful bacteria throughout your body.

Yet, the key is recognizing these situations and understanding that modern medicine excels in urgent, emergency, and acute care. But, once this crisis passes, it is important to seek healing in a way that respects the body's natural processes, rather than relying solely on medical interventions to mask symptoms. I tell my patients that I work with the body, I do not force it into submission. When you have a

long-term type of illness, it is always better to work with the body to move with it, as it is always trying to keep you, the owner, in a state of health.

Section 4: The Power of Healing Naturally

The real power of healing comes when we recognize that prevention and long-term well-being are best achieved through a lifestyle that supports the body's natural processes. This is where you will find that The Savage Diet comes into play.

Ancestral healing methods – such as proper nutrition, physical activity, stress management, and sleep –

are the foundations for a thriving body. For many chronic conditions like autoimmune disorders, digestive issues, and hormonal imbalances, modern medicine often relies on drugs that manage the symptoms, but do not address the root cause. This is again, the quick fix mentality, whereas, The Savage Diet offers a holistic approach to these problems, eating whole foods and focusing on the nutrient-dense foods that mimic our ancestors' way of eating.

For instance, instead of relying on medications for inflammation, we can embrace natural antiinflammatory foods such as wild-caught fish, leafy greens and bone broth. Will you get an instantaneous result? No. However, over the course of time, this way of eating will decrease your overall body inflammation (body burden), and you won't have any inflammation present. You will most likely reduce any extra weight, and decrease the amount of visceral fat present, which will decrease the burden on your joints and decrease the work your organs have to do.

Reducing or completely eliminating processed foods can benefit your body in countless ways. You will automatically decrease the toxic burden on your system. Additionally, by simply removing those types of

"foods," you will also reduce the amount of inflammation in your body. While in medical school, I had a professor tell us that it was not necessary to put a patient on a specific diet to lose weight or bring about positive changes in their health; all we had to do was assess the diet and remove "the Junk." This is very true. I have been recommending The Savage Diet to patients for years, and many of those who have followed it have lost weight and improved their well-being, as noted in the review section. I have also encountered many people so engrossed in the Standard American Diet, that they simply do not understand a whole-food diet.

Section 5: Integrating Both Worlds: A Balanced Approach To navigate the waters of modern medicine as a Savage is to understand that both worlds have value. It's about knowing when to lean into modern solutions, but also when to turn inward, trusting your body's ability to heal with the right support.

1. Preventive Care with Ancestral Foundations:

I believe that prevention is the ultimate form of self-care. To focus on nutrient-dense whole foods, and movement that mimics our ancestral ways, all mental practices that promote calm and clarity, avoiding the toxins that are so rampant in our society today. By building a resilient body, you can often prevent the need for many of the chronic medications that modern medicine tends to prescribe. I utilize all the conveniences of modern medicine, to find where my patient is at. For example, when I see a patient, I am always looking to have them age well. What does that mean? It means that I am also thinking of their bone health, their hormones, and their stress etc.

This is because, while the body is forgiving, and we expect a lot from it, over the course of time, it will react to too much of anything.

2. Informed Decision-Making:

When faced with a health concern, take the time to understand your options. Research your condition, question your healthcare provider about the causes of your symptoms, and seek out solutions that work in harmony with your body's natural systems. If a doctor prescribes

medication, inquire about natural alternatives that could complement or reduce the need for pharmaceuticals. If you encounter a healthcare provider who dismisses your concerns, or brushes over your questions, then you have found someone who does not recognize that there are other options besides a medication, and I would look for someone more in tune with looking at the whole picture. One of the easiest treatments is a pill. It makes life so much easier for the doctor. However, when you look at natural medicine, you have no end to the different modalities you can use to help your patient from a much deeper level.

3. Restoring Balance:

When modern medicine does become necessary—whether through surgery, antibiotics, or other treatments—ensure you are also taking steps to restore balance. A nourishing diet, movement, and stress-reducing practices should be part of your healing journey to help your body bounce back as quickly and completely as possible. Whenever I prescribe an antibiotic for someone, I always follow it up with a probiotic, and encourage the patient to eat with different whole-food prebiotics and probiotics.

4. Mindful Approach to Modern Technologies:

While modern technologies like MRIs, surgeries, and blood tests can be invaluable, it is crucial to not become overly reliant on them. Use these tools as they are intended: as instruments that provide insight and solutions, not as the sole determinant of your health.

Section 6: The Path Forward: Empowerment Through Knowledge The way forward is one of balance and empowerment. As a savage navigating modern medicine, you must take an active role in your health, becoming informed and confident in your decisions. Embrace the technologies and advancements that modern medicine has to offer, but do so with the understanding that true healing begins from within. Use the wisdom of the ancients and the resources of modern medicine to create a life that is vibrant, balanced, and free from unnecessary dependence. I tell my patients that "I do not want them to be sitting in a wheelchair, peeing in their pants, or drooling on their chin". This is probably a crude way to say it, but I want my patients to be independent through their lives. I do not want them to have to be in a nursing home, or have their children take care of them.

Ultimately, navigating modern medicine as a savage is about choosing the right path at the right time—

one that honors your body's innate wisdom while also embracing the power of modern science to provide safety and support when needed. In this way, you can live a life of health, rooted in the ancestral ways yet empowered by the advancements of today. Hippocrates (considered the father of medicine), is famous for saying; "Let food be thy medicine and medicine be thy food". I could not say it any better. Choose your food wisely.

This is the cornerstone of reclaiming control over our health and well-being. The Savage Diet is meant to be empowering, it is not just about learning to eat differently, but it is also about understanding why these choices are vital and how they work in harmony with our bodies. When we are armed with knowledge, whether it is about nutrition, our body's natural healing mechanisms, or the way our modern society impacts our health – we gain the power to make informed decisions that align with our ultimate goal.

Health and longevity.

When we focus on nutrient-dense foods and their bioavailability, we know that this is what our bodies were designed to thrive on to maintain the balance within. We have discussed how the Standard American Diet is very deficient in nutrients, and how processed foods that we are exposed to daily have contributed to a range of negative effects on our bodies.

Chronic inflammation is linked to many diseases, the high sugar content, unhealthy fats and artificial additives increase the production of inflammatory molecules, which can disrupt the body's natural immune response.

Part VI: The Savage vs Modern Diets

Chapter 11: Your Savage Journey

Section 1: Diet Wars: Keto, Paleo, and Mediterranean—Which Best Supports Your Gut?

The gut is often called the "second brain" due to its profound impact on physical and mental health. It is home to trillions of microorganisms, including bacteria, fungi, viruses, and archaea, which form the gut microbiome. This ecosystem plays a pivotal role in digestion, nutrient absorption, and immune function. A balanced and diverse microbiome is essential for efficient digestion, as it helps break down complex foods, produce beneficial compounds like short-chain fatty acids, and protect the gut lining from harmful pathogens. Moreover, the microbiome communicates directly with the immune system, influencing inflammatory responses, immune cell activity, and the body's defense against infections. Disruptions to the microbiome can lead to gastrointestinal issues, weakened immunity, and increased susceptibility to chronic diseases. So, where do the different diets come into play, and how do they affect your microbiome?

There are many similarities in the diets, and they are all good and can be used at any time because, for the most part, you eliminate all toxins, sugars, and in some of the diets, sometimes the grains. Notice that I said "for the most part." No matter what diet it is, there is always a section on how to make a very sweet treat by adding some Stevia, milk, or some type of grain. Our ancestors occasionally enjoyed treats, perhaps some berries during certain times of the year, and they had honey if they were fortunate; it all depended on where they were on the planet. This is The Savage Diet, which includes few treats made from natural products.

Section 2: Gut Health and Keystone Microbes

Gut health is at the heart of overall wellness, influencing everything from digestion to immune function, and even mood regulation. The gut is a complex ecosystem of trillions of microorganisms—they range from bacteria to fungi and viruses—and work together to maintain a balance that supports these vital functions. The human gut microbiome plays an essential role in breaking down food, absorbing nutrients, defending against pathogens, and regulating immune responses. So, a diverse and balanced microbiome is the foundation for a healthy digestive system and immune function, making it essential for maintaining optimal health. In this chapter, we will explore the significance of gut health, the importance of building a diverse microbiome with fiber-rich foods, and how fermented foods and natural probiotics can play a critical role in supporting and maintaining gut health on The Savage Diet. I feel like the bane of my existence because I always harp on the importance of the Gut daily to my coworkers and anyone who will listen, but I feel very strongly, that we ignore our gut health so much that it is fighting back at us. I feel our microbiome is not evolutionarily adept at handling all of what we have thrown at it over the course of the last one hundred years, and it is fighting the only way that it can. By symptoms. Our body tells us, when there is something wrong, we just never listen.

Section 3: The Importance of Gut Health for Immunity and Digestion
The gut microbiome is essential for a range of bodily functions. These microbes help break down food, extract nutrients, and even synthesize vitamins and fatty acids that are critical for health. The gut's health is directly linked to the body's ability to digest food, absorb nutrients, and regulate metabolism. Beyond digestion, the gut microbiome is deeply involved in immune function. It is currently estimated that up to 70% of the body's immune system is located in the gut, and the microbiome interacts

with the immune system, influencing the production and regulation of immune cells and antibodies. A nice, healthy,

balanced microbiome helps to maintain a well-functioning immune system, reducing the likelihood of infections and chronic diseases.

In contrast, disruptions to the gut microbiome—caused by factors such as poor diet, stress, antibiotics, or environmental toxins—can lead to dysbiosis, which is a state of microbial imbalance. Dysbiosis can result in various digestive issues, including bloating, gas, and constipation, as well as more severe conditions like inflammatory bowel disease (IBD), irritable bowel syndrome (IBS), and even autoimmune diseases. A disrupted microbiome can also weaken the immune system, making the body more susceptible to infections, inflammation, and chronic conditions such as allergies and autoimmune disorders.

So, maintaining a healthy gut is essential for digestion and the body's ability to fight disease, as well as inflammation regulation. The role of the diet in shaping the gut microbiome cannot be understated, it is so important to nourish it with foods that support microbial diversity and balance. In my daily interactions with patients, as they explain to me their diet, I can tell immediately that they have no diversity in the gut.

Section 4: Fermented Foods and Natural Probiotics in the Savage Diet Fermented foods are another cornerstone of a healthy gut microbiome. These foods are rich in live beneficial bacteria, or probiotics, which help restore balance to the gut and promote optimal digestion.

Probiotics are microorganisms that, when consumed in adequate amounts, confer a health benefit to the host—helping to restore the gut's microbial balance, improve digestion, and support immune function.

Fermented foods like kimchi, sauerkraut, kefir, yogurt (for those who tolerate dairy), kombucha, and fermented vegetables contain live probiotics that can support a healthy gut.

Fermentation is when bacteria and yeasts break down sugars and starches in food, creating beneficial compounds such as lactic acid and other organic acids. These fermented foods contain both probiotics and bioactive compounds, enzymes, and antioxidants that support gut health and enhance the body's ability to absorb nutrients. Regular consumption of fermented foods can help increase the population of good bacteria in the gut, reduce the growth of harmful bacteria, and improve the gut's overall microbial diversity. For The Savage Diet, incorporating fermented foods is a good way to restore balance to the gut microbiome. These foods are nutrient-dense, full of beneficial bacteria, and can help enhance digestion while improving immune function. Kimchi, sauerkraut, and pickled vegetables are great additions to the diet, providing beneficial probiotics and also supporting the immune system's ability to fight off infections.

Additionally, dairy-free fermented foods such as coconut yogurt or water kefir can be excellent alternatives for those avoiding dairy.

Fermented foods not only improve the gut's microbial health but, also enhance the bioavailability of nutrients from the rest of the diet. For example, fermenting vegetables can increase the availability of minerals like calcium and magnesium, making them easier for the body to absorb. Incorporating fermented foods into The Savage Diet aligns with its focus on whole, unprocessed foods, enhancing digestion, boosting the immune system, and promoting microbial diversity. Whether it's through a serving of fermented vegetables, a cup of kombucha, or a small portion of kimchi, these foods can serve as a daily ally for gut health. Many of my patients make their own Kefir, Kombucha, and Kimchi, and I applaud them, as they are taking a stand for their own health.

Section 5: Gut Diversity and Brain Health

Gut diversity plays a crucial role in brain health through a connection known as the gut-brain axis, which is the bidirectional communication between the gut and the brain, involving the Vagus nerve, which is cranial nerve X. This complex system involves a combination of pathways, including the nervous system, the immune system, and biochemical signaling. We will discuss below how gut diversity specifically benefits brain health.

Certain gut microbes are involved in the synthesis of neurotransmitters, which are chemicals that help transmit signals in the brain. As an example, Serotonin, which is a neurotransmitter that is associated with mood regulation, is predominantly produced in the gut (about 90% of it). The diversity of gut bacteria can influence the production and balance of serotonin, which affects mood, anxiety, and depression and GABA (Gamma-Aminobutyric Acid), is an inhibitory neurotransmitter that promotes relaxation and reduces anxiety, and it is also produced by certain gut microbes.

So, a more diverse gut microbiome supports the balanced production of these neurotransmitters, which leads to better emotional regulation, reduced stress, and improved mental clarity.

A diverse microbiome helps to keep inflammation in check. Chronic low-grade inflammation is a known contributor to various brain-related disorders, such as depression, anxiety, and neurodegenerative diseases like Alzheimer's. A well-balanced gut microbiome will help to reduce systemic inflammation by producing short-chain fatty acids (SCFAs) such as butyrate, which have anti-inflammatory effects. These SCFAs can cross the blood-brain barrier and reduce neuroinflammation, thus supporting brain function and mental health, this was discussed earlier.

Balance immune responses, as about 70% of the immune system resides in the gut. A healthy microbiome can promote a stronger and more regulated immune response, preventing excessive inflammation that could negatively impact brain health.

Section 6: Gut Microbes and the Stress Response

The gut microbiome influences the body's stress response by regulating the hypothalamic-pituitaryadrenal (HPA) axis, which governs the release of stress hormones like cortisol. So, imbalances in gut diversity can lead to an overactive stress response, increasing vulnerability to mental health disorders like anxiety and depression. On the other hand, a diverse microbiome helps maintain a balanced HPA axis and reduces the harmful effects of chronic stress.

Section 7: Cognitive Function and Memory

Gut bacteria influence the brain's ability to process information, form memories, and regulate emotions.

Research has shown that a more diverse microbiome can enhance cognitive function by influencing brain plasticity (the brain's ability to adapt and form new connections). The SCFAs produced by gut bacteria, particularly butyrate, have been shown to promote brain-derived neurotrophic factor (BDNF), which is involved in learning, memory, and cognitive health.

The gut bacteria also reduce the risk of neurodegenerative diseases, as a diverse gut microbiome can support mechanisms that protect brain cells from damage. On the other hand, imbalances in the microbiome have been linked to conditions like Alzheimer's disease and Parkinson's disease. I tell my patients daily, that gut diversity has a direct impact on mental health. A healthy microbiome helps modulate the gut-brain signaling pathways, which influence mood, anxiety levels, and overall emotional well-being. And a diverse microbiome is associated with lower levels of depression, anxiety, and stress. It can regulate the blood-brain barrier to protect the brain from harmful pathogens and toxins, promoting better overall brain health and emotional stability.

Section 8: Gut Health and the Blood-Brain Barrier

The blood-brain barrier (BBB) is a protective layer that shields the brain from harmful substances. A healthy, diverse microbiome can help maintain the integrity of the blood-brain barrier, preventing harmful substances from crossing into the brain that might otherwise lead to neurodegenerative diseases, chronic inflammation, or mental health disorders. It supports brain detoxification, as some gut bacteria help process and eliminate toxins from the body, reducing the load on the brain.

A diverse gut microbiome not only aids digestion but, it also profoundly affects brain health. This is by influencing neurotransmitter production, regulating inflammation, enhancing cognitive function, and maintaining a balanced stress response, gut diversity supports optimal brain function and mental wellbeing. The more diverse your gut bacteria, the better your body can manage mental health, protect against brain degeneration, and regulate emotional responses.

Part VII: The Scientific Backbone

Chapter 12: The Evidence Supporting the Savage Diet

Section 1: The Evidence

The principles of the Savage Diet are deeply rooted in evolutionary biology and nutritional science, which reflects on how humans are biologically designed to thrive on whole, nutrient-dense foods. In this chapter we are going to explore the scientific foundation of the Savage Diet, so I will demonstrate the health benefits of ancestral eating patterns.

As we venture into the world of The Savage Diet, I believe it's important to understand this concept. I want to emphasize that this is not a diet to follow; it is a lifestyle to embrace. I believe that in order to maintain our health, we absolutely must take control of our own outcome.

Our evolutionary history has shaped how our bodies process and respond to food. From the beginning of our known time on earth, at least 2.5 – 3 million years ago, we primarily survived on a diet of animal protein, vegetables, fruits, nuts, and seeds. As we moved through history by thousands and millions of years, this diet provided all the essential nutrients that our bodies required for survival and optimal function. Modern diets by contrast, have shifted dramatically over the past 200 years, largely due to the industrialization of agriculture, and the introduction of refined grains and processed foods. All for the sake of convenience and money, especially this past century.

All of the scientific research has shown that our ancestors were not only well-adapted to the huntergatherer lifestyle, but this diet shaped their genetic makeup. Our bodies evolved to digest and utilize whole, unprocessed foods. The shift to modern, processed diets, I believe, has led to a host of chronic diseases. Of course, the most common is obesity, heart disease and diabetes.

Studies on the genetic evolution of humans highlight that our metabolism is suited for a diet high in protein, healthy fats, and low in refined carbohydrates. Our bodies must have protein and fats, but there is no requirement for carbohydrates, as we produce our own through a process called gluconeogenesis, but today we typically get carbohydrates from exogenous sources, which is contributing to the obesity crisis. Through gluconeogenesis we produce the glucose necessary for fueling the brain and muscles; this is done through non-carbohydrate sources like proteins and fats. This typically occurs in the liver where amino acids (from protein) and glycol (from fats) are converted into glucose.

The Savage Diet is focused on high-quality protein and healthy fats, unlike processed carbohydrates, which can spike blood sugar levels and contribute to insulin resistance. The protein and fats provide for sustained energy, essential fatty acids and support for hormone production.

The benefits of consuming higher amounts of animal protein are significant as animal proteins are considered "complete" proteins, meaning they contain all of the essential amino acids our bodies require.

I hesitate to mention this because I do not want everyone to go and buy out the shelves of meat at the

grocery store. We don't have the quality of meat that I want at the big box grocery store. I hunt around and find a local source that has elk, bison, or beef, but are all grass-fed and finished. Why do I do this?

Because I have to make a choice on what I feel is best for me and my family. With that choice also comes the reality of what I can afford to buy. I say you need protein, and you do, however; we share a steak at home, and rarely have meat again for a couple of days. I will make fish, or chicken or do a salad with shrimp.

A study that was published in The American Journal of Clinical Nutrition found that a diet high in proteins, can lead to greater fat loss and preservation of muscle mass during weight loss. Research consistently demonstrates that higher protein intake can increase metabolism, improve satiety and support the preservation of lean muscle mass during weight loss. That being said, there is a balanced state, if you tip the scales with too little or not enough, then your body will react in some way. When you have an intake of protein your body breaks it down into amino acids, which is then used for various functions like building muscles, enzymes and hormones. However, if you consume more protein than your body needs for these purposes, the excess amino acids can be converted into glucose through Gluconeogenesis. This will raise blood sugar levels, and if it is not used for energy, then it can be stored as fat.

Healthy fats, such as fatty fish and grass-fed animals, help maintain our levels of Omega-3 fatty acids.

They are essential for improving insulin sensitivity, reducing chronic inflammation, and are considered cardioprotective. These fats play a crucial role in keeping us full and satisfied, making it easier to regulate our appetite and avoid overeating. Research from The Journal of Clinical Endocrinology and Metabolism suggests that higher-fat diets can improve fat oxidation and promote a healthier weight. Our bodies need fat. I understand that when you visit your doctor and your cholesterol is close to 199, it may feel like you're being encouraged—or I've heard from my patients, frightened—into starting a statin drug. Many do, but try to stay calm and remember you are in control of your health. There are very few reasons I can think of that would not allow you time to change your diet to lower your cholesterol to levels acceptable to your doctor. However, I will also mention that our guidelines for cholesterol have changed over the years.

Remember that if you eat grass-fed beef, the cow is not producing any additional cholesterol beyond what it gets from its grass diet. The meat has very little marbling, if any at all. The diet is the main difference between the types of beef; this significantly affects the fatty acid composition and the types of cholesterol they contain. While both types of beef can provide essential nutrients, their nutritional quality, particularly regarding cholesterol and fat content, differs.

Grass-fed beef has a healthier Omega-3 to Omega-6 fatty acid ratio, as they consume a diet rich in grass and forage, which is high in mega-3. As we discussed previously, Omega-3s are known to reduce inflammation, improve heart health, and support brain function. Grass-fed beef also typically contains higher levels of conjugated linoleic acid (CLA) and Omega-3 fatty acids, which have been linked to various health benefits, including a reduced risk of cardiovascular disease.

Conventionally raised beef are typically fed grains like corn and soy, which are high in Omega-6 fatty acids. While we discussed that omega-6 fats are essential for the body, an imbalance between Omega-6

and Omega-3 fats, (i.e., consuming too much Omega-6) can promote inflammation, which is a risk factor for heart disease and other chronic conditions. Because of the higher ratio of Omega 6 to Omega 3, grain-fed beef is less beneficial for overall health, with more risk factors overall.

There is another aspect that I would like to cover as well. Cows have a unique digestive system consisting of four compartments: the rumen, the reticulum, the omasum, and the abomasum. The digestive tract is specifically adapted for breaking down fibrous plant material, such as grass, hay and other roughage. The rumen, the largest compartment, is home to billions of microbes that help break down the fiber in grass through fermentation. This allows the cows to extract the nutrients from plant fibers that would be indigestible to humans or monogastric (one stomach) animals. Grains on the other hand, are much easier to digest than fibrous plants. They are starchy and contain simple sugars, feeding them in excess disrupts the natural fermentation process in the rumen. In other words, the cows are not

designed to process such high concentrations of starch, which can lead to several health issues for the cows. It disrupts several things, but let me suffice it to say, it disrupts their microbiome that weakens the cow's immune system, making it more vulnerable to infections and chronic health conditions. Hmm, that sounds familiar, doesn't it?

Grain feeding causes cows to grow quickly, and in addition to the antibiotics and female hormones they are given, this comes at a cost to their long-term health. Cows tend to accumulate more fat than lean muscle and, again, more Omega-6 than Omega-3.

Additionally, grain feeding can affect the nutritional quality of the meat itself.

The modern diet is centered around eating grains, especially the refined ones – along with sugar and highly processed foods. These foods are associated with health issues, including all of the regular diseases of obesity, type 2 diabetes, heart disease, and gut health imbalances. The research supporting the elimination of grains, sugars and processed foods is extensive and compelling. As we have discussed previously, studies that show gluten found in wheat, barley and rye can cause inflammation and digestive issues in individuals with celiac disease and non-celiac gluten sensitivity. Even in people without these conditions, gluten can disrupt the gut health by promoting leaky gut, and then eventually leading to systemic inflammation. Studies published in The American Journal of Gastroenterology has found that gluten-free diets can improve gut health and reduce symptoms of irritable bowel syndrome (IBS), bloating and discomfort

Section 2: Evolutionary Biology and the Case for Ancestral Diets The relationship between the human genome and environmental factors is central to understanding our nutritional needs. Over millions of years, we evolved in response to our environment, which meant adapting to available food sources in various climates and geographic regions. The ancestral diet, rooted in the hunter-gatherer lifestyle, primarily consisted of animal proteins, fats, and certain plant-based foods, which helped early humans thrive.

As our ancestors migrated across diverse landscapes, their diets shifted in response to local resources, from the nutrient-rich foods found in coastal areas to the leaner meats and foraged plants in colder climates. This evolution shaped the human genome, with genetic traits developing to optimize the digestion of specific food types, such as the ability to process starches or tolerate dairy products, depending on environmental conditions.

Environmental factors like climate changes, migration, and the availability of food shaped how our ancestors developed biochemically. The human body evolved to rely on fats for energy, with brain development and overall survival relying heavily on animal-based nutrients, including proteins, fats, and specific vitamins and minerals like Omega-3 fatty acids and zinc.

Carbohydrates played a minimal role in the diet, as early humans adapted to primarily burning fat and protein for fuel, an ability that still remains part of our metabolic system today, although we have changed this somewhat by our reliance of simple carbohydrates and all of the processed foods we eat. Early human health was defined by a nutrient-dense diet that helped prevent many of the prevalent chronic diseases in the modern world.

In contrast, the advent of agriculture and industrialization disrupted this balance. The modern diet, laden with processed foods and sugars, bears little resemblance to the ancestral diet and is poorly suited to our genetic makeup. This mismatch between our evolutionary biology and the foods we now consume has contributed to the rise in chronic health issues. By returning to a more ancestral way of eating—focused on high-quality fats, proteins, and unprocessed vegetables—we can optimize our health and align our nutrition with the evolutionary needs that shaped our species. The wisdom of our ancestors offers a powerful tool for reclaiming our health in the modern world, and embracing this approach can help us avoid the health pitfalls of today's industrialized food system.

Section 3: Benefits of Whole, Nutrient-Dense Foods

Numerous studies confirm that whole foods—such as vegetables, fruits, lean proteins, and healthy fats—

offer higher concentrations of vitamins, minerals, and antioxidants compared to processed foods.

Research shows that diets rich in these foods reduce the risk of chronic diseases. Vegetables like leafy greens are high in vitamins A, C, and K, while fruits such as berries provide essential antioxidants that combat oxidative stress. When you eat whole foods, you have the whole enchilada in one package. It will have all of the essential vitamins, minerals, fiber and antioxidants that are crucial for the body to function optimally.

Processed foods, on the other hand, often lack fiber and essential nutrients while being high in sugars, refined carbohydrates, and unhealthy fats. Whole foods encourage better digestive health. Fiber helps regulate bowel movements, prevent constipation and feed beneficial gut bacteria, which promotes a healthier, more balanced gut microbiome.

Whole foods tend to be more filling and satisfying compared to processed foods. As I have said, I recommend avoiding foods like all grains, legumes, dairy and refined sugars, which are considered part of the modern processed diet. When you eliminate grains, which can sometimes cause digestive issues, and it usually does, it is just that we do not know it, simply because we dismiss the signs of bloating, gas and discomfort.

Part VIII: The Rest of the Savage Life

Chapter 13: Bringing Your Savage Life Together

Section 1: The Art of Being Mindful

When we are fully present and engaged in the moment, and without judgment. Cultivating awareness of your thoughts, emotions, bodily sensations, and the surrounding environment. As we practice a holistic lifestyle, I believe mindfulness serves as a tool to harmonize the mind, body, and spirit, fostering a deeper connection with yourself and the world around you. When we are mindful, it encourages intentional living.

It helps individuals align their actions and choices with their values and well-being. I believe being mindful transformed our lives 20,000 years ago. Taking intentional control of their mindfulness as a way of life, although I am sure they did not label it as such. Their very survival depended on being in the present moment, they were very attuned to their environment and deeply connected to it. As they were foraging for plants, herbs, and berries, they remained very aware of their surroundings. They paid attention to the movement of the environment, always listening to the sounds around them. If the birds were singing or if they stopped singing, they became acutely aware there may be danger lurking nearby. The hunters practiced acute focus, awareness and patience in tracking animals over long distances. So, every sound, footprint or broken branch was carefully noted, fostering an intimate connection with their surroundings.

Because they lived in harmony with nature's rhythms, they observed the moon's cycles, the changes in weather, and seasonal shifts. This awareness dictated their movements, food sources, and survival strategies. Being mindful of their environment allowed them to conserve their resources, to avoid predators and work with, not against nature. Walking was not just a means of getting from one place to another; it was a deeply embodied practice. As they walked, they could feel how their bodies moved, they could sense when it was time to rest and adapt their pace based on their energy levels and the demands of the journey itself. They remained mobile through the long winter months, as they had to follow the food sources as they migrated to different, but not always warmer, climates.

They practiced (unknowingly) mindful movement. Whether it was by walking, climbing or running, it was intentional and graceful. The study of fossil footprints gives us some insight into the walking mechanics of early humans. For example, footprints found at Laetoli, Tanzania, dating back 3.6 million years show evidence of fully upright, human-like bipedal walking. The observations of modern hunter-gatherer societies such as those of the Kalahari desert, reveal that mobility is central to their way of life. Their mobility involves a pattern, where groups will aggregate into larger units and split up periodically or seasonally, indicating a deliberate and meaningful approach to movement and planning.

Walking and movement were not just physical acts, but expressions of mindfulness that balanced survival needs and every step was a reflection of their awareness, adaptability and respect for the environment that sustained them.

Section 2: Meditation

Meditation is a practice that focuses the mind and often includes techniques such as deep breathing, visualization, or mantra repetition. It is a process of training attention and awareness to achieve a mentally clear, emotionally calm, and stable state. Meditation is a restorative practice within a holistic lifestyle, allowing the mind to reset and rejuvenate. It supports emotional resilience, reduces stress, and enhances focus, thereby complementing physical health and spiritual growth.

Our early human ancestors probably did not meditate in the same manner as we do today, but they likely engaged in meditative or contemplative practices as part of their survival and spiritual activities. In comparing our ancestors of 20,000 years ago to modern-day hunter-gatherers, we know they gathered for rituals around the fire or their sacred sites. A ceremony that involved rhythmic chanting, drumming or dancing, which induced trance-like meditative states. These practices likely helped them connect with the spiritual world, in turn strengthening their bonds within their community and processing their emotions.

Shamanic traditions that are present in many cultures involve long periods of stillness, silence, or focused visualization, which is very similar to our own techniques that many of us use today.

Living in close harmony with nature, our ancestors spent extended periods of time observing their surroundings in silence.

Section 3: Join me 20,000 years ago under the Silent Stars...

The fire crackled softly, its warm glow casting dancing shadows on the nearby trees. Ekon sat crosslegged on the cool earth, his spear resting beside him. Tonight, the hunt was done, the tribe fed and the world was quiet. He tilted his head back, his dark eyes tracing the infinite tapestry of the stars above.

Each tiny light shimmered and pulsed, as though deep in silent conversation. Ekon had learned from the elders that these stars were the spirits of ancestors, watching over them, guiding their steps. As he observed them, he felt their silent wisdom seep into his being, calming the restless thoughts of the day.

The night sang with a symphony of life. To his right, leaves rustled softly— a small family of deer grazed cautiously beneath the moonlight, their movements graceful and deliberate, as though they too, understood the sacred stillness of the moment. A soft hoot broke the silence, and Ekon turned his gaze upward to spot a great horned owl perched high in a tree, its large eyes mirroring his own curiosity. Ekon breathed deeply, the scent of the damp earth and pine filling his lungs. He closed his eyes for a moment, focusing on the sounds around him-the chirping of crickets, the distant howl of a wolf, the gentle whisper of the wind through the trees. Each sound blended into a harmonious rhythm, a song of the wild that resonated with his heartbeat.

Opening his eyes, he looked up at the stars in all of their grandeur, his gaze fell upon a constellation the elders called "The Hunter", its pattern forever etched in his memory. It reminded him of his own place in the great cycle of life, not as a conqueror of nature, but a part of it. The stars above, the animals around him, and the fire by his side, they were all connected, woven into the same fabric of existence.

Ekon reached down, his fingers brushing against the cool soil. He whispered a silent gratitude to the earth for its gifts, to the stars for their guidance, and to the creatures for their companionship. The owl hooted again as if in response, and Ekon smiled softly to himself. In the stillness, he felt profound peace.

This was his meditation, his connection to his ancestors, the earth, and the universe. Under the silent stars, Ekon was not just a hunter, not just a man. He was a thread in the vast, eternal web of life. And for tonight that was enough.

Mindfulness and meditation serve as foundational elements of a holistic lifestyle rather than merely as stress-relief techniques. They enable people to handle life's challenges, enhance self-awareness, and cultivate a profound sense of peace and purpose. In

229

the Savage Lifestyle framework, these practices are vital for reconnecting with ancestral rhythms, navigating contemporary stress, and embracing the transformative power inherent in this way of life.

- Mental health benefits of mindfulness practices.

- Techniques for meditation, breathing, and stress reduction.

- Aligning your mind with your body for holistic health.

Section 4: Music and Drums

One of the things I remember with vivid detail and exceptional clarity is growing up as a child in northern Wyoming. Each year, we would host the rodeo in my town and always invited the Native American tribes that lived nearby, as there are several reservations in the surrounding areas. I remember lying in bed and hearing their drums playing all night long. To this day, I can lie back and feel the beat of the hide drums pulsating in sync with my heartbeat.

All over the world, people use drums not only to communicate, but through them, they tell stories and dance and have different ceremonies.

For spiritual and religious ceremonies drums were used in ancient rituals to communicate with the divine or invoke spiritual power. In many early cultures, drumming was seen as a way to connect with gods, spirits, and ancestors. The rhythmic beats were thought to bridge the gap between the physical world and the spiritual realm.

In ancient shamanistic traditions, drums were often used to induce trance-like states, enabling shamans to journey to other realms or communicate with the spirit world. The repetitive, rhythmic sound of the drum helped to alter consciousness and helped facilitate spiritual experiences. This practice can still be seen in modern-day indigenous cultures.

Drums were used during rites of passage such as births, coming-of-age ceremonies, marriages, and funerals. The rhythm of the drum would mark significant moments in an individual's or community's life cycle, reinforcing identity, culture, and the connection to ancestors.

Drumming was also a tool for marking changes in the seasons, which were critical to ancient agricultural societies. Seasonal festivals often involved drumming as a way to celebrate harvests, honor deities associated with the earth, or seek blessings for the coming cycle.

The use of drums has held a sacred and central role in human history, from their use in spiritual ceremonies, communication, and social cohesion to their significance in war and personal identity. For ancient peoples, including those from 20,000 years ago, the drum was not just an instrument—it was a vital tool for shaping culture, fostering unity, and transcending the human experience through rhythm and sound.

Testimonials

Jessica – Reversing Type 2 Diabetes and Finding Energy

Background: Jessica, 52, had been living with type 2 diabetes for five years, relying heavily on insulin.

She had struggled with weight gain, fatigue, and blood sugar fluctuations, and her doctor suggested that if things didn't improve, her health could further deteriorate.

Testimonial:

When Jessica adopted The Savage Diet, she focused on eliminating processed sugars and refined grains while incorporating healthy fats and lean proteins into her meals. She embraced intermittent fasting, gradually extending her fasting window. Within two months, her blood sugar stabilized to the point where Dr. Mendoza titrated her insulin down, which was further reduced and ultimately discontinued. Over the next year, she lost 30 pounds, felt energized, and noticed improvements in her mental clarity.

"I feel free for the first time in years. No more afternoon crashes or constant cravings. It's like a fog has lifted."

Michael – Conquering Heart Disease and Weight Issues

Background: At 48, Michael had dangerously high cholesterol levels and was warned he needed to take statins to avoid a heart attack. He had tried other diets but found them hard to sustain. With a family history of heart disease, he knew he needed a permanent lifestyle change.

Testimonial:

Michael committed to The Savage Diet by prioritizing grass-fed meats, fish, olive oil, and leafy greens while avoiding industrial seed oils and processed foods. He also integrated a weekly fasting protocol.

After six months, his cholesterol profile was within normal limits, with an increase in HDL and a decrease in LDL. He lost 25 pounds and built strength through functional workouts aligned with the diet's principles.

"What surprised me was how sustainable it became. I didn't just lose weight—I gained control over my health."

Sophia – Tackling Autoimmune Issues and Chronic Fatigue

Background: Sophia, 34, had been struggling with Hashimoto's thyroiditis and chronic fatigue for years.

She experienced joint pain, brain fog, and daily exhaustion, which impacted her ability to work and enjoy life.

Testimonial:

Sophia followed the Savage Diet's autoimmune protocol, eliminating inflammatory foods like grains, legumes, and dairy. She incorporated bone broth, fermented vegetables, and fatty fish to promote gut healing. Within four months, her energy levels returned, her joint pain decreased, and her thyroid function improved significantly.

"It felt like my body was fighting me before, but now we're finally on the same team. The diet gave me my life back."

David – A Lifelong Struggle with Weight and Emotional Eating
Background: David, 41, had tried every diet imaginable, from low-fat to keto, without lasting success. His weight fluctuated, and emotional eating habits made it difficult to maintain long-term change. He felt hopeless and frustrated.

Testimonial:

The mindset shift of The Savage Diet clicked for David. He embraced the holistic approach, combining mindfulness practices with a whole-food-based diet. David found that removing processed foods naturally reduced his cravings. Over the course of a year, he lost 50 pounds, but more importantly, he developed a healthy relationship with food.

"It's not just about food anymore—it's about feeling good. I stopped seeing meals as rewards and started seeing them as fuel."

Elena – Thriving Through Menopause

Background: Elena, 55, found herself struggling with menopause symptoms, including hot flashes, mood swings, and weight gain. She had tried supplements and hormone therapy, but nothing seemed to work long-term.

Testimonial:

By adopting The Savage Diet, Elena focused on healthy fats, lean proteins, and nutrient-dense vegetables. She also used intermittent fasting to manage her energy levels. Within three months, she noticed fewer hot flashes, improved sleep, and emotional stability.

"Menopause no longer feels like a curse—it's just another phase of life. The Savage Diet helped me feel strong and balanced."

Jane B. - Healing

Dr. Dianna Mendoza is a caring and thorough doctor, very personable. She took schooling as an allopathic doctor, then as a naturopath, so you get the better of both worlds. She is very much a "let's get to the bottom of this" kind of person. Dr. Dianna is interested in your healing, not just covering the symptoms with medication.

Kim T. -

I have never actually written a Review for a product or a service but this time, I cannot keep this to myself.

I am 55 yrs old, battled with weight (and bad eating habits) most of my life along with committing to a work-out program, and have been suffering through bouts of sleeplessness & menopause for 6-7 years. I tried old and trusted diets & work-out routines but with my recent hormone imbalances, nothing worked.

As a matter-of-fact, I gained 10 more pounds over the holidays!!

During a routine visit to my Chiropractor and seeing her weight-loss, I inquired as to how in the world she was doing this! I joked that maybe she just bought a larger sized 'Scrubs'? LOL...then she handed me a card for Dr. Mendoza. At that point, my life changed. After doing it my way for 50 years with little to no (lasting) success, I had to let go of everything I 'thought' I knew about a healthy life-style and open my mind to a better way, a smarter way, a Way that works. In the first week, I lost 5 pounds - in the first month, I have lost 11 pounds, and a total of 10 inches. At this rate, I will see my goal in a matter of a couple of months.

I look so forward to my check-ups with Dr. M which are filled with reviewing my food journal, exercise log (Caroline Girvan is our favorite!), exchanging recipes (modified to suite my new habits), lots of laughing, and trouble-shooting small issues that come along (how to replace a food item with a healthier choice).For the first time in my life I cannot wait to get on the scale or be measured! We also upgraded all of my old supermarket-grade supplements to a better quality and added a couple.

Dr. M's patience with me and her amazing listening skills have helped me to feel heard which, in turn, makes me feel empowered. We are now branching out into thermal-imaging in lieu of a standard mammogram, meditation, and myofascial therapy to take my health quality to another level. Breaking old bad habits can be hard but with Dr. Mendoza's help, it gets easier plus after seeing (and feeling) the results, even easier! My new way of Life is so exciting and has sparked my creativity on cooking, working out and now a new wardrobe coming soon! Thank You Dr. M!

Just M. - Health

I believe when good service is rendered, it should be recognized. That being said, I would add, Covid has created many obstacles to true health care. Having had to work around the medical restriction I personally found it difficult to find any one in Cottonwood willing to work WITH me. Then I met the people at Casket Mountain, and I was blown away. This group of ladies are not only remarkable, but from a relationship standpoint, they are friendly, generous with their time, compassionate, and exceptional in every way. Ones relationship with their physicians, and staff is paramount to ones overall health. You will find it all at Casket Mountain. Their prices are extremely reasonable, as well. After 2 years of working on my health issues, I know I am on the right track, my health over the last 3 months working WITH Casner is remarkably improved, to the extent that even friends and acquaintances have noticed. It would be well

worth the time to contact them if you are not satisfied with the treatment you are currently receiving. To say I love my Dr, is an understatement, 5 stars seem hardly enough!

Mark V.

I contacted Dr. Mendoza because I was tired of the experience going to normal doctors and them prescribing a pill to mask the underlying issues. I needed help with controlling inflammation in my body and I made a great choice in finding Dr. Mendoza. Since I've started visiting with her through carefully prescribed blood screenings and allergy testing for both food and substances, I'm happy to say that I'm on my way back to amazing health.

After my first meeting with Dr. Mendoza and her prescribing a simple diet in the interim, I lost almost 7 lb in one week just by removing certain foods. Visiting a naturopathic practitioner doctor was the best thing I ever did. Additionally, I also saw Dr. Mendoza for IV supplement treatments, which have sent my energy levels through the roof.

Thank you, Dr. Mendoza, for everything you've helped me accomplish with my body!

R.K

Dr. Dianna Mendoza is the most professional, intelligent and intuitive naturopath that I have worked with. I initially reached out after months of being treated for recurring/ongoing sinus infection. From that first visit, I could see she was thinking as she was speaking. She was very thoughtful in her words and advice.

I am very impressed by her perseverance in dealing with my issue.

Through a combination of acupuncture, a physical procedure and medication, she finally brought me relief.

I appreciate that she was always very conscious of costs involved with either tests or medications. I'm continuing to work with her on ongoing preventative medicine and weight loss. I have no doubt, with her advice, I will succeed with both goals.

Notes

1. Ancestral Diet and Evolutionary Biology:

o Cordain, L., & Konner, M. (2009). The Paleo Diet: Lose Weight and Get Healthy by Eating the Foods You Were Designed to Eat. Wiley.

o Eaton, S. B., & Konner, M. (1985). Paleolithic Nutrition: A Consideration of Its Nature and Current Implications. New England Journal of Medicine, 312(5), 283-289.

o Lindeberg, S. (2010). Food and Western Disease: Health and Nutrition from an Evolutionary Perspective. Wiley-Blackwell.

2. The Role of Protein, Fats, and Carbohydrates in Human Evolution: o Hawkes, K., & O'Connell, J. F. (2004). Human Diet and Evolutionary Nutrition. In Essays in Human Evolution, University of Chicago Press. o

Mann, N., & Cummings, J.

(2009). The Role of Fat and Protein in Human Evolution. Evolutionary Anthropology, 18(5), 206-220.

3. Gut Health and Keystone Microbes:

o Bäckhed, F., et al. (2005). The Human Gut Microbiome and Its Role in Health and Disease. Nature, 473(7347), 204-211.

o Cho, I., & Blaser, M. J. (2012). The Human Microbiome: At the Interface of Health and Disease. Nature Reviews Genetics, 13(4), 260-270.

o Sonnenburg, J. L., & Sonnenburg, E. D. (2019). The Good Gut: Taking Control of Your Weight, Your Mood, and Your Long-Term Health. Penguin Press.

4. Inflammation and Disease Prevention:

o Spector, T. D. (2015). The Diet Myth: The Real Science Behind What We Eat. Flatiron Books.

o Calder, P. C. (2006). Polyunsaturated Fatty Acids and Inflammation. Proceedings of the Nutrition Society, 65(3), 335-342. o

Jørgensen, K. A., et al. (2017). Inflammatory

Markers in Chronic Disease. Journal of Internal Medicine, 282(3), 235-246.

5. The Modern Diet vs. Ancestral Eating:

o Harris, M. (2010). The Ancient Diet: How Modern Eating Habits Are Undermining Your Health. McGraw-Hill.

o Lindeberg, S. (2010). Food and Western Disease: Health and Nutrition from an Evolutionary Perspective. Wiley-Blackwell.

o Pollan, M. (2008). In Defense of Food: An Eater's Manifesto. Penguin Press.

6. Chronic Disease and the Role of Diet in Reversal:

o Campbell, T. C., & Campbell, T. M. (2004). The China Study: The Most Comprehensive Study of Nutrition Ever Conducted and the Startling Implications for Diet, Weight Loss, and Long-term Health. BenBella Books.

o Esselstyn, C. B., et al. (2009). Prevention and Reversal of Coronary Artery Disease: An Update. Journal of Family Practice, 58(6), 275-283.

o Ornish, D. (1998). Dr. Dean Ornish's Program for Reversing Heart Disease. Ballantine Books.

7. Nutritional Science and Metabolic Health:

o Taubes, G. (2007). Good Calories, Bad Calories: Fats, Carbs, and the Controversial Science of Diet and Health. Anchor Books.

o Ludwig, D. S. (2002). The Glycemic Index: A Physiological Basis for Carbohydrate Exchange. American Journal of Clinical Nutrition, 76(1), 5-56.

8. Mindfulness and Meditation in Health:

o Kabat-Zinn, J. (2005). Wherever You Go, There You Are: Mindfulness Meditation in Everyday Life. Hyperion.

o Goleman, D. (2013). Focus: The Hidden Driver of Excellence. HarperCollins. o Siegel, D. J. (2010). The Mindful Brain: Reflection and Attunement in the Cultivation of WellBeing. W.W. Norton & Company.

References

Eaton, S. B., & Konner, M. (1985). "Paleolithic Nutrition: A Consideration of Its Nature and Current Implications." *New England Journal of Medicine*, 312(5), 283-289.

DOI:10.1056/NEJM198501313120505

Cordain, L., et al. (2005). "Origins and Evolution of the Western Diet: Health Implications for the 21st Century." *American Journal of Clinical Nutrition*, 81(2), 341-354.

DOI:10.1093/ajcn.81.2.341

Aune, D., et al. (2017). "Fruit and Vegetable Intake and the Risk of Cardiovascular Disease, Total Cancer, and All-Cause Mortality." *International Journal of Epidemiology*, 46(3), 1029-1056. DOI:10.1093/ije/dyw319

Micha, R., et al. (2017). "Association Between Diet Quality and Mortality in the USA."

JAMA, 317(9), 912-924. DOI:10.1001/jama.2017.0941

Liu, R. H. (2013). "Health Benefits of Fruit and Vegetables Are from Additive and Synergistic Combinations of Phytochemicals." *American Journal of Clinical Nutrition*, 78(3), 517S-520S. DOI:10.1093/ajcn/78.3.517S

Monteiro, C. A., et al. (2018). "Ultra-Processed Foods and the Need to Reframe Dietary Guidelines." *Public Health Nutrition*, 21(1), 50-56. DOI:10.1017/S1368980018001367

Ludwig, D. S., & Ebbeling, C. B. (2018). "The Carbohydrate-Insulin Model of Obesity."

Journal of the American Medical Association, 319(3), 209-210.

DOI:10.1001/jama.2017.20061

Hallberg, S. J., et al. (2018). "Effectiveness and Safety of a Novel Care Model for the Management of Type 2 Diabetes at One Year." *Diabetes Therapy*, 9(2), 583-612.

DOI:10.1007/s13300-018-0373-9

Seidelmann, S. B., et al. (2018). "Dietary Carbohydrate Intake and Mortality." *The Lancet Public Health*, 3(9), e419-e428. DOI:10.1016/S2468-2667(18)30135-X

Calder, P. C., et al. (2011). "Omega-3 Fatty Acids and Inflammatory Processes." *Nutrition Reviews*, 69(9), 535-549. DOI:10.1111/j.1753-4887.2011.00467.x Koh, A., et al. (2016). "The Microbiome and Metabolic Health." *Annual Review of Physiology*, 79(1), 481-502. DOI:10.1146/annurev-physiol-021115-105415 Monteiro, C.

A., Moubarac, J.-C., Cannon, G., Ng, S. W., & Popkin, B. (2013). Ultraprocessed products are becoming dominant in the global food system. *Obesity Reviews*, 14(S2), 21-28.

Mozaffarian, D., Rosenberg, I., & Uauy, R. (2018). History of modern nutrition science—

implications for current research, dietary guidelines, and food policy. *BMJ Global Health*, 3(1), e000513.

Mattson, M. P., Longo, V. D., & Harvie, M. (2017). Impact of intermittent fasting on health and disease processes. *Ageing Research Reviews*, 39, 46-58.

Patterson, R. E., & Sears, D. D. (2017). Metabolic effects of intermittent fasting. *Annual Review of Nutrition*, 37, 371-393.

Warburton, D. E., & Bredin, S. S. (2017). Health benefits of physical activity: A systematic review of current systematic reviews. *Current Opinion in Cardiology*, 32(5), 541-556.

Park, B.-J., Tsunetsugu, Y., & Miyazaki, Y. (2010). The physiological effects of Shinrin-yoku (taking in the forest atmosphere or forest bathing): Evidence from field experiments in 24 forests across Japan. *Environmental Health and Preventive Medicine*, 15(1), 18-26.

Kabat-Zinn, J. (2015). Mindfulness-based stress reduction. *Clinical Psychology: A Guide to Evidence-Based Practice*, 393-400.

Holt-Lunstad, J., Smith, T. B., & Layton, J. B. (2010). Social relationships and mortality risk: A meta-analytic review. *PLoS Medicine*, 7(7), e1000316.

Sonnenburg, E. D., & Sonnenburg, J. L. (2019). *The Good Gut: Taking Control of Your Weight, Your

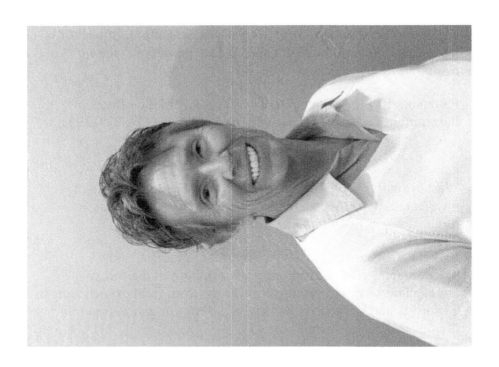

"Discover the Diet That Ignites Your Primal Power and Reverse
Chronic Disease"

Modern Diets are failing us. The very foods we're told to eat are
the ones contributing to the rise in chronic diseases, fatigue and
weight gain. But what if the secret to vibrant health was hidden in
our ancestors' diet as well as their way of life?

The Savage Diet is a groundbreaking approach that taps into the
ancestral wisdom our bodies are craving. It's not just about eating
differently- it is about reclaiming your health, energy and strength
by rediscovering how humans were meant to nourish themselves.

By combining nutrient-dense whole foods, mindful movement, and ancient wisdom, this book will teach you how to reverse diseases, optimize your gut health, and build the body and life you deserve. This isn't about a fad diet- *The Savage Diet* is a lifestyle transformation that empowers you to reclaim the savage strength within.

Inside, you will learn:

How to unlock the healing power of real, whole foods.

Why modern diets make us sick, and how to break free from them.

Practical steps to improve gut health, boost energy, and lose weight naturally.

Proven strategies to reverse chronic disease and restore balance to your body.

As a Naturopathic Physician and a passionate advocate for ancestral living, I've seen firsthand the extraordinary power of *The Savage Diet* to heal, transform, and uplift lives. Now it is your turn. Are you ready to discover the strength within you? Are you ready to transform your life?

It is time to awaken the savage within and embrace a new path to health. The journey starts here.

Document Outline

-
-
-
-
-
-
-
-
-
-
-
-
-
-
-
-
-
-
-
-
-
-
-
-
-
-

-
-
-
-
-
-
-
-
-
-
-
-
-
-
-
-
-
-
-
-

Made in the USA
Las Vegas, NV
20 February 2025

18440314R00144